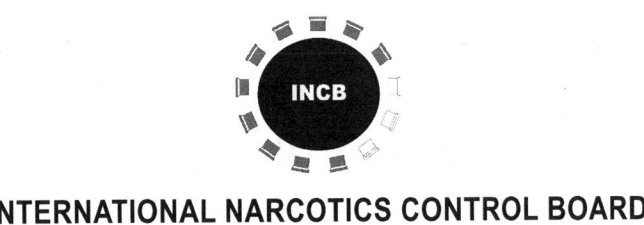

INTERNATIONAL NARCOTICS CONTROL BOARD

Precursors
and chemicals frequently used in the illicit manufacture of narcotic drugs and psychotropic substances

Report of the International Narcotics Control Board for 2016 on the Implementation of Article 12 of the United Nations Convention against Illicit Traffic in Narcotic Drugs and Psychotropic Substances of 1988

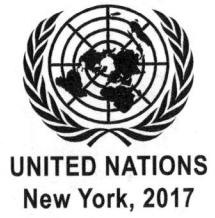

UNITED NATIONS
New York, 2017

E/INCB/2016/4

UNITED NATIONS PUBLICATION
Sales No. E.17.XI.4
ISBN: 978-92-1-148290-4
eISBN: 978-92-1-060067-5

Print ISSN: 2411-8664
Online ISSN: 2411-8672

© United Nations: International Narcotics Control Board, January 2017. All rights reserved worldwide.
Publishing production: English, Publishing and Library Section, United Nations Office at Vienna.

Foreword

It is my pleasure to present the International Narcotics Control Board's 2016 report on precursors, its first annual report on precursors following the thirtieth special session of the General Assembly, on the world drug problem.

INCB welcomes the joint commitment of Member States, expressed in the outcome document of the special session, to addressing and countering the world drug problem. Specifically, INCB welcomes their commitment to preventing and countering the diversion of precursors and pre-precursors for illicit use. The Board is pleased to see that Member States have extended their commitment to include pre-precursors, substitute and alternative precursors and chemicals used in the illicit manufacture of new psychoactive substances, i.e., chemicals which require cooperation beyond the letter of the United Nations Convention against Illicit Traffic in Narcotic Drugs and Psychotropic Substances of 1988. The Board is also pleased to note the emphasis on voluntary partnerships and cooperation with relevant industries, an area to which it attaches great importance, as highlighted in the Board's 2015 report on precursors.

Throughout the outcome document, Governments also emphasize the importance of and the need for enhanced information-sharing, multilateral operational cooperation, including joint investigations, and the use of existing tools and cooperation mechanisms, in order to identify, disrupt and dismantle organized criminal groups that are involved in, among other things, the diversion of precursors.

The present report provides Governments with the Board's latest analysis of the functioning of the international precursor control system and a comprehensive overview of the most recent precursor trends and challenges, in accordance with the Board's mandate under the 1988 Convention. In our conclusions, we address a number of overarching concerns that emerge from our analysis of this year's data and information. An area previously addressed that has increased in importance is the vulnerability of the global precursor control systems in periods of political instability in a number of countries and entire regions.

The present report also picks up on the concerns of the special session's outcome document and provides a thematic focus on the prevention of chemical diversion beyond regulatory controls, namely the role of law enforcement, and a call to overcome competing interests, compartmentalization and the mentality that considers seizures to be the ultimate goal of an intervention, rather than focusing on identifying and disrupting the sources and criminal groups behind attempts to obtain the necessary chemicals.

On behalf of the Board, I therefore wish to invite all Governments and interested international and regional organizations to work with each other, the Board and its secretariat, to maximize the effectiveness of precursor control, encompassing the continuum from regulatory to law enforcement measures, as a preventive element of an integrated and balanced strategy to counter the world drug problem.

Werner **Sipp**

President of the International
Narcotics Control Board

Preface

The United Nations Convention against Illicit Traffic in Narcotic Drugs and Psychotropic Substances of 1988 provides that the International Narcotics Control Board shall submit a report annually to the Commission on Narcotic Drugs on the implementation of article 12 of the Convention and that the Commission shall periodically review the adequacy and propriety of Tables I and II of the Convention.

In addition to its annual report and other technical publications (on narcotic drugs and psychotropic substances), the Board has prepared its report on the implementation of article 12 of the 1988 Convention in accordance with the following provisions contained in article 23 of the Convention:

1. The Board shall prepare an annual report on its work containing an analysis of the information at its disposal and, in appropriate cases, an account of the explanations, if any, given by or required of Parties, together with any observations and recommendations which the Board desires to make. The Board may make such additional reports as it considers necessary. The reports shall be submitted to the [Economic and Social] Council through the Commission which may make such comments as it sees fit.

2. The reports of the Board shall be communicated to the Parties and subsequently published by the Secretary-General. The Parties shall permit their unrestricted distribution.

Contents

	Page
Foreword	iii
Preface	v
Explanatory notes	ix

Chapter

			Page
I.	Introduction		1
II.	Action taken by Governments and the International Narcotics Control Board		1
	A.	Scope of control	1
	B.	Adherence to the 1988 Convention	1
	C.	Reporting to the Board pursuant to article 12 of the 1988 Convention	2
	D.	Legislation and control measures	3
	E.	Submission of data on licit trade, uses and requirements	4
	F.	Annual legitimate requirements for imports of precursors of amphetamine-type stimulants	5
	G.	Pre-export notifications and utilization of the PEN Online system	6
	H.	Activities and achievements in international precursor control	8
III.	Extent of licit trade in precursors and the latest trends in precursor trafficking		9
	A.	Substances used in the illicit manufacture of amphetamine-type stimulants	10
	B.	Substances used in the illicit manufacture of cocaine	21
	C.	Substances used in the illicit manufacture of heroin	24
	D.	Substances used in the illicit manufacture of other narcotic drugs and psychotropic substances	27
	E.	Solvents and acids used in the illicit manufacture of various narcotic drugs and psychotropic substances	28
	F.	Substances not in Table I or Table II of the 1988 Convention that are used in the illicit manufacture of other narcotic drugs and psychotropic substances or substances of abuse not under international control	30
IV.	Prevention of chemical diversion beyond regulatory controls: the role of law enforcement		32
V.	Conclusions		34
Glossary			38

Annexes*

		Page
I.	Parties and non-parties to the 1988 Convention, by region, as at 1 November 2016	41
II.	Annual legitimate requirements for ephedrine, pseudoephedrine, 3,4-methylenedioxyphenyl-2-propanone and 1-phenyl-2-propanone, substances frequently used in the manufacture of amphetamine-type stimulants	47
III.	Substances in Tables I and II of the 1988 Convention	53
IV.	Use of scheduled substances in the illicit manufacture of narcotic drugs and psychotropic substances	54

---

* The annexes are not included in the printed version of the present report but are available in the CD-ROM version and in the version on the website of the International Narcotics Control Board (www.incb.org).

V.	Treaty provisions for the control of substances frequently used in the illicit manufacture of narcotic drugs and psychotropic substances	58
VI.	Regional groupings...	59
VII.	Submission of information by Governments pursuant to article 12 of the 1988 Convention (form D) for the years 2011-2015...	60
VIII.	Seizures of substances in Tables I and II of the 1988 Convention, as reported to the International Narcotics Control Board, 2011-2015	65
IX.	Submission of information by Governments on licit trade in, uses of and requirements for substances in Tables I and II of the 1988 Convention for the years 2011-2015.............	100
X.	Governments that have requested pre-export notifications pursuant to article 12, paragraph 10 (a), of the 1988 Convention	107
XI.	Licit uses of the substances in Tables I and II of the 1988 Convention	112

Figures

I.	Timeline of form D submissions by States parties to the 1988 Convention, 2011-2015.......	2
II.	Seizures of ephedrine and pseudoephedrine reported by Governments on form D, 2011-2015	11
III.	Number of laboratories dismantled in the Islamic Republic of Iran, 2008-2015..............	12
IV.	Seizures of ephedrine and pseudoephedrine raw materials reported on form D by the Government of India, 2006-2015	14
V.	Seizures of APAAN communicated through PICS and reported on form D, 2012-2016	17
VI.	Seizures of chemicals associated with illicit methamphetamine manufacture reported on form D by Mexico, 2009-2015...	19
VII.	Seizures of potassium permanganate reported by Governments on form D, 2011-2015	22
VIII.	Seizures of potassium permanganate and its precursors, as reported on form D by Colombia, 2000-2015...	23
IX.	Seizures of sodium metabisulfite, as reported on form D, 2008-2015	24
X.	Seizures of acetic anhydride (in litres), as reported on form D, 2010-2015.................	25
XI.	Seizures of acetic anhydride, as reported on form D by Afghanistan, 2010-2015............	26
XII.	Seizures of ammonium chloride reported on form D by Afghanistan and other countries, 2011-2015	27
XIII.	Seizures of solvents in Table II and non-scheduled acetate solvents, as reported on form D by Colombia, 2006-2015...	29

Table

States parties failing to report as required under article 12, paragraph 12, of the 1988 Convention, 2015...	3

Maps

1.	Governments that have registered with the Pre-Export Notification Online system and those that have invoked article 12, paragraph 10 (a), of the 1988 Convention, requiring pre-export notification for selected substances (As at 1 November 2016)	6
2.	Governments registered with and that are using the Precursors Incident Communication System (as at 1 November 2016)...	9

Explanatory notes

The boundaries and names shown and the designations used on the maps in this publication do not imply official endorsement or acceptance by the United Nations.

The designations employed and the presentation of the material in this publication do not imply the expression of any opinion whatsoever on the part of the Secretariat of the United Nations concerning the legal status of any country, territory, city or area or of its authorities, or concerning the delimitation of its frontiers or boundaries.

Countries and areas are referred to by the names that were in official use at the time the relevant data were collected.

Multiple government sources of data were used to generate the present report, including the information provided each year on form D (information on substances frequently used in the illicit manufacture of narcotic drugs and psychotropic substances), notifications via the Pre-Export Notification Online (PEN Online) system, the Precursors Incident Communication System (PICS) and other official communications with competent national authorities. Unless otherwise specified, data provided on form D are referred to by the calendar year to which they apply; the cut-off date for reporting the data is 30 June of the following year. The reporting period for data from the PEN Online system and PICS is from 1 November 2015 to 1 November 2016, unless otherwise specified. In cases in which PEN Online data are used for multiple years, calendar years are used. Additional information was also provided through regional and international partner organizations, as indicated in the report.

Reference to "tons" is to metric tons, unless otherwise stated.

The following abbreviations have been used in the present report:

ANPP	4-anilino-*N*-phenethyl-4-piperidine
APAA	*alpha*-phenylacetoacetamide (2-phenylacetoacetamide)
APAAN	*alpha*-phenylacetoacetonitrile
GBL	*gamma*-butyrolactone
GHB	*gamma*-hydroxybutyric acid
INCB	International Narcotics Control Board
INTERPOL	International Criminal Police Organization
MDMA	3,4-methylenedioxymethamphetamine
3,4-MDP-2-P	3,4-methylenedioxyphenyl-2-propanone
NPP	*N*-phenethyl-4-piperidone
P-2-P	1-phenyl-2-propanone
PCP	phencyclidine
PEN Online	Pre-Export Notification Online
PICS	Precursors Incident Communication System

Summary

As in previous years, the International Narcotics Control Board (INCB) notes an overall discrepancy between what is indicated by available information on precursors and their sources, and the wide availability of illicitly manufactured drugs.

This is true for seizures of both internationally controlled methamphetamine precursors, such as ephedrine and pseudoephedrine, and their substitutes, in East and South-East Asia, in the context of the large and growing methamphetamine market in that region. It is also true for acetic anhydride and other chemicals required to process opium into morphine and subsequently into heroin: seizures of precursors used to manufacture heroin in South-East Asia are virtually non-existent; seizures in Afghanistan have declined at a year-on-year rate of 50 per cent for the fourth consecutive year; and countries in Central Asia that share borders with Afghanistan have not reported any seizures for more than 15 years. By contrast, an increase in the reported seizures in Iran (Islamic Republic of) and Pakistan is beginning to reveal a more realistic picture of acetic anhydride trafficking in the region.

Whereas INCB has previously alerted countries about the absence of precursor information relating to the Near and Middle East, a region known for large-scale seizures of so-called "captagon" tablets, recent seizures in Lebanon and the prevention of a diversion attempt involving a company in the Syrian Arab Republic have now shed some light on the situation. Similarly, it is now clear that methamphetamine in Mexico is increasingly being illicitly manufactured from benzaldehyde, a chemical that is not under international control but which has been controlled in Mexico since January 2016. In 2016, for the first time, an illicit methamphetamine manufacturing operation in Nigeria used the same manufacturing method as in Mexico, suggesting that the country, as well as other countries in Africa, continue to be targeted by criminal organizations for precursor trafficking.

The significant seizures of ephedrine and pseudoephedrine in India and Nepal in 2016 highlighted once again the need for better national controls and understanding of legitimate manufacturing methods, domestic distribution channels and the operators and their roles in the national market. The same applies to chemicals used for the manufacture of cocaine, as the information available suggests that most seizures of potassium permanganate, the key oxidizing chemical, continued to be traceable to diversion from domestic distribution channels or illicit manufacture from pre-precursors, such as was found in cases in Colombia.

A number of previously reported non-scheduled "designer" chemicals to substitute for amphetamine-type stimulants precursors continued to be seized, such as esters and salts of 1-phenyl-2-propanone (P-2-P) methyl glycidic acid and 3,4-methylenedioxyphenyl-2-propanone (3,4-MDP-2-P) methyl glycidic acid; and new ones emerged, especially in Europe, a development that appears to be related in part to the placing of *alpha*-phenylacetoacetonitrile (APAAN) under international control in 2014. Similarly, following the international scheduling of mephedrone, a synthetic cathinone that had been previously considered a "new psychoactive substance", there has been an increasing number of incidents, mainly in Europe, involving precursors of that substance, which are not under international control.

The other region where non-scheduled substances constituted an important share of chemical seizures was South America, especially with regard to non-scheduled solvents, which were seized in volumes exceeding those of scheduled solvents. Increasing amounts of seizures of sodium metabisulfite and calcium chloride, two chemicals used to increase the efficiency of cocaine processing, indicate increasingly greater levels of organization of the related illicit activities and continued high levels of recycling of solvents.

With respect to the functioning of the international precursor control system, INCB is pleased to note the continued increase in the number of countries requesting pre-export notifications by invoking article 12, paragraph 10 (a), and the increasing use of Pre-Export Notification Online (PEN Online) and the Precursors Incident Communication System (PICS), the basic tools made available by the Board to support Governments in their efforts against chemical diversion. At the same time, the present report puts a special focus on the law enforcement component of precursor control, an area that is not being used to its full potential to prevent chemical diversion and which was also addressed in broader terms in the outcome document of the thirtieth special session of the General Assembly on the world drug problem, held in April 2016.

I. Introduction

1. The International Narcotics Control Board (INCB) monitors Governments' control over precursor chemicals and assists Governments in preventing the diversion of such chemicals from licit into illicit channels, pursuant to the provisions of the United Nations Convention against Illicit Traffic in Narcotic Drugs and Psychotropic Substances of 1988.[1] The present report has been prepared pursuant to the provisions of that Convention.

2. Substantive reporting begins in chapter II, which provides statistical data and other information on action taken by Governments and the Board pursuant to article 12 of the 1988 Convention. Those data are drawn from a number of sources, including the following: form D; the Pre-Export Notification (PEN Online) system; the Precursors Incident Communication System (PICS); the operational results achieved under Project Prism and Project Cohesion, which are the international initiatives addressing chemicals used in the illicit manufacture of, respectively, amphetamine-type stimulants, and cocaine and heroin; and official national reports on the drug and precursor control situation.

3. Chapter III provides information on the extent of legitimate trade in individual precursor chemicals; on major trends in trafficking in and illicit use of those chemicals; on relevant cases of suspicious and stopped shipments; on diversions or attempted diversions of those chemicals from legitimate trade; and on seizures of those chemicals, including clandestine laboratories.

4. As has been the practice since 2011, one precursor-related theme is addressed in greater depth in the report. In this year's report, chapter IV explores the role of precursor law enforcement in preventing diversions, including the diversion of non-scheduled substitute chemicals.

5. Specific recommendations and conclusions are highlighted throughout the report to facilitate concrete actions to be taken by Governments to prevent diversion. Overall conclusions are presented in chapter V.

6. Annexes I-X to the report provide updated statistics and practical information to assist competent national authorities in carrying out their functions. The annexes are not included in the printed copies of the present report but are available in the electronic version (CD-ROM) and on the INCB website.

II. Action taken by Governments and the International Narcotics Control Board

7. The present chapter provides information on action taken by Governments and the Board since its 2015 report on precursors.

A. Scope of control

Initiation of procedures for the inclusion of two precursors of fentanyl in Table I of the 1988 Convention

8. In October 2016, the Government of the United States of America notified the Secretary-General of a proposal to place N-phenethyl-4-piperidone (NPP) and 4-anilino-N-phenethyl-4-piperidine (ANPP), two precursors of fentanyl and of a few "designer" fentanyls, in Table I of the 1988 Convention. Pursuant to the procedure set out in article 12, paragraph 3, of that Convention, the Secretary-General invited Governments' comments concerning the notification and supplementary information which might assist the Board in establishing an assessment and assist the Commission on Narcotic Drugs in reaching a decision.

B. Adherence to the 1988 Convention

9. As at 1 November 2016, the 1988 Convention had been ratified, acceded to or approved by 189 States and formally confirmed by the European Union (extent of competence: article 12). As there have been no changes since the publication of the Board's 2015 report on precursors (see annex I), there continue to be nine States — five in Oceania, three in Africa and one in West Asia — that have yet to become parties to the 1988 Convention.[2] **The Board urges the nine States that have yet to become parties to the 1988 Convention to implement the provisions of article 12 and accede to the Convention without further delay.**

---

[1] United Nations, *Treaty Series*, vol. 1582, No. 27627.

[2] Equatorial Guinea, Kiribati, Palau, Papua New Guinea, Solomon Islands, Somalia, South Sudan, State of Palestine and Tuvalu.

C. Reporting to the Board pursuant to article 12 of the 1988 Convention

10. Article 12, paragraph 12, of the 1988 Convention requires States parties to submit annually to INCB aggregated information pertaining to the previous year, on: seizures of substances in Tables I and II of the 1988 Convention and, when known, their origin; any substance not included in Table I or II which is identified as having been used in illicit manufacture of narcotic drugs or psychotropic substances; and methods of diversion and manufacture. Such information is to be submitted in form D at the latest by 30 June of the following year, although INCB encourages an earlier submission (30 April) to facilitate its analysis and ensure sufficient time for any necessary clarification of information provided.

11. As at 1 November 2016, 120 States parties had submitted form D for 2015 (see annex VII for details); of those, 71 States parties submitted form D on time, by 30 June 2016, the highest rate in five years. In past form D reporting cycles, a number of countries submitted their forms after the final cut-off date, with the result that those forms could not be considered in the annual report for the respective year (see figure I). Similar to last year, 6 per cent of form D submissions were made using older versions of form D, thus providing an incomplete set of information. **Governments are reminded to use the latest version of form D, which is available, in the six official languages of the United Nations, on the INCB website, and submit it within the requested timeline to facilitate the Board's analysis of the world precursor situation.**

Figure I. Timeline of form D submissions by States parties to the 1988 Convention, 2011-2015

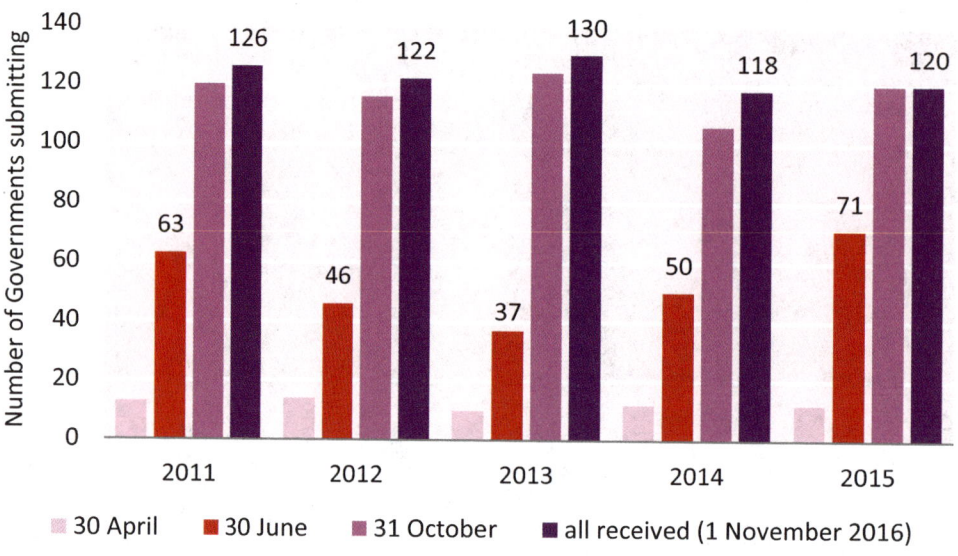

12. Sixty-four States parties to the 1988 Convention failed to report to the Board the information for 2015.[3] Of those, two States parties have never submitted form D, and 23 States parties have not done so in the past five years (see table). Kenya resumed submission after failing to submit form D for four years; Burundi submitted form D for the first time. **The Board thanks those Governments that have provided a complete form D and wishes to remind all other Governments that the submission of form D is mandatory under article 12, paragraph 12, of the 1988 Convention and that submission of blank forms or of partial information continues to impact the Board's analysis of regional and global precursor patterns and trends.**

13. In 2015, while 83 States parties provided information on seizures of substances in Table I or Table II of the 1988 Convention on form D (for details on the reported seizures of those substances, by region, see annex VIII), only 45 parties provided information of operational relevance with a view to identifying weaknesses and emerging trends and preventing future diversions, such as substances not included in Tables I and II (43 Governments, or 36 per cent of all 120 submitting States parties) and information on methods of diversion and illicit manufacture (24 Governments, or 20 per cent). While such information is often available in media reports, reported in national reports or in official conference presentations and sometimes communicated through PICS, it

---

[3] The Holy See, Liechtenstein, Monaco and San Marino did not furnish form D separately as their data are included in the reports of France, Italy and Switzerland.

is too often not reported on the annual form D. Therefore, INCB wishes to commend Governments that shared operational details and remind all other Governments effecting seizures or encountering alternate substances to provide all relevant details of such seizures on form D, in particular, information on origin, where known, and methods of diversion and illicit manufacture.

Table. States parties failing to report as required under article 12, paragraph 12, of the 1988 Convention, 2015

Algeria	Fiji	Niger[a]
Angola[a]	Gabon[b]	Nigeria
Antigua and Barbuda[a]	Gambia	Niue
Bahamas[a]	Grenada[a]	Paraguay
Barbados	Guinea[a]	Qatar
Belize	Guinea Bissau	Saint Kitts and Nevis[a]
Botswana[a]	Iraq	Samoa
Burkina Faso Cambodia	Kuwait	Sao Tome and Principe
Cameroon	Lesotho[a]	Serbia
Central African Republic[a] Chad	Liberia[a]	Seychelles
	Libya[a]	Sierra Leone[a]
Comoros[a]	Luxembourg	Suriname[a]
Congo[a]	Malawi[a]	Swaziland[a]
Cook Islands	Maldives	The Former Yugoslav Republic of Macedonia[a]
Côte d'Ivoire	Marshall Islands[b]	
Cuba	Mauritania[a]	Timor-Leste
Djibouti[a]	Mauritius	Togo
Dominica[a]	Micronesia	Tonga[a]
Dominican Republic	Mozambique	Vanuatu
Eritrea	Namibia	Yemen
	Nauru	Zambia
	Nepal	

Note: See also annex VII.
[a] Government that failed to submit form D for any year during the period 2011-2015.
[b] Government that has never submitted form D.

D. Legislation and control measures

14. In accordance with the provisions of article 12 of the 1988 Convention and the relevant resolutions of the General Assembly, the Economic and Social Council and the Commission on Narcotic Drugs, Governments are requested to adopt and implement national control measures to effectively monitor the movement of precursor chemicals. In addition, Governments are also requested to further strengthen existing precursor control measures should any weaknesses be identified. The following changes in control measures have been brought to the attention of INCB since the publication of its last report on precursors.

15. In November 2015, Australia passed an amendment to the Criminal Code Act 1995, removing the element of "intent to manufacture" from offences relating to the importation of "border-controlled precursors". The element required, for the offence to apply, that a person who imported or exported a "border-controlled precursor" had done so either with the intent to use it to illicitly manufacture a controlled drug or had the belief that another person intended to use the substance to illicitly manufacture a controlled drug ("intent to manufacture" element). However, there had been significant difficulties in proving the intention or belief of the persons, especially if they were part of a larger operation and deliberately operated with limited knowledge about how their actions fitted into the broader criminal enterprise.

16. In China, the ninth amendment of the Chinese criminal law became effective on 1 November 2015, adding two new precursor-related offences to the criminal law, namely, illicit

manufacture of precursor chemicals and illicit transportation. The amendment also increased the maximum sentencing for precursor-related crimes, including a provision for the confiscation of property and for punishing as conspiracy the illicit manufacture of drugs.

17. Following the international scheduling of *alpha*-phenylacetoacetonitrile (APAAN) effective 6 October 2014, Canada added APAAN, its salts, isomers, and salts of isomers to part 1 of schedule VI of the Controlled Drugs and Substances Act and to the schedule to the Precursor Control Regulations (PCR) on 24 February 2016; in Norway, APAAN was scheduled on 19 March 2016.

18. In June 2016, the Canadian senate passed a bill to amend the Controlled Drugs and Substances Act to include six chemicals, often key intermediary products, used in the manufacture of fentanyl, namely, NPP, 4-piperidone, norfentanyl, 1-phenethylpiperidin-4-ylidene phenylamine, *N*-phenyl-4-piperidinamine, as well as the salts of the aforementioned substances, and propionyl chloride; the last-mentioned has been included in the INCB limited international special surveillance list of non-scheduled chemicals since 2007.

19. Effective 21 September 2016, European Commission Delegated Regulation (EU) 2016/1443, which amended Regulation (EC) No. 273/2004 of the European Parliament and of the Council and Council Regulation (EC) No. 111/2005, added chloroephedrine and chloropseudoephedrine (and their optical isomers), two "designer" precursors of methamphetamine, to the scheduled substances list (category 1). The amendment subjects these substances to the strictest measures provided for under the European Union harmonized control and monitoring measures.

20. In response to the international scheduling of APAAN, the 2017 edition of the World Customs Organization's *Harmonized System Nomenclature*, which entered into force effective 1 January 2017, includes a new harmonized system code number for the separate identification of APAAN. In addition, new code numbers were also introduced to improve the monitoring and control of pharmaceutical preparations containing ephedrine, pseudoephedrine or norephedrine. The amendments were made at the request of INCB.

21. As in the past, updated information about individual national systems of authorizations applied to imports and exports of substances in Tables I or II of the 1988 Convention, as well as to additional substances under national control, is available on the secure website of INCB, for use by competent national authorities. The INCB information package on the control of precursors is updated whenever new information is made available to INCB.

22. In April 2016, the thirtieth special session of the General Assembly on the world drug problem concluded with the adoption of an outcome document in which Member States reconfirmed their joint commitment to addressing and countering the world drug problem. In response, the Government of Thailand, in a letter to INCB, informed INCB of its request for all Governments to pay more attention to the control of precursor chemicals and cooperate in the interdiction of precursors to prevent them from entering areas in which illicit drug manufacture takes place. **INCB welcomes the outcome document of the thirtieth special session of the General Assembly and the commitment of Governments to the core principles of international precursor control, including the monitoring of international trade through the PEN Online system, operational cooperation under Project Prism and Project Cohesion and through PICS, and public-private partnerships. In relation to the appeal of the Government of Thailand, INCB invites all countries and territories to further strengthen their cooperation with the Board and with each other on all matters related to the implementation of their treaty obligations under article 12 of the 1988 Convention.**

E. Submission of data on licit trade, uses and requirements

23. Knowing the legitimate market and understanding and recognizing the nature and extent of regular trade, uses and requirements is a prerequisite for identifying unusual trade patterns and preventing diversions. To that end, and pursuant to Economic and Social Council resolution 1995/20, INCB requests information on licit trade in, use of, and requirements for substances in Tables I and II of the 1988 Convention on form D. Provision of those data is on a voluntary and confidential basis and allows INCB to help Governments to prevent diversion by identifying patterns of suspected illicit activity.

24. As at 1 November 2016, the Governments of 115 States parties had provided information on licit trade in substances in Tables I and II of the 1988 Convention, and 111 had furnished data on licit uses of and/or requirements for one or more of the substances in Tables I and II of the 1988 Convention (see annex IX). The Governments of Burundi, Kenya and Rwanda submitted licit trade data for the first time in the five-year period. **INCB commends those Governments that provide comprehensive licit trade data**

for substances in Tables I and II of the 1988 Convention and wishes to encourage all other Governments to provide such data, confidentially if so desired, to help to understand the patterns of regular trade and licit requirements in order to facilitate the identification of suspicious activity and prevent diversion of those substances.

F. Annual legitimate requirements for imports of precursors of amphetamine-type stimulants

25. For more than a decade, Governments have been providing estimates of annual legitimate requirements for imports of precursors of amphetamine-type stimulants to the Board, pursuant to Commission on Narcotics Drugs resolution 49/3, entitled "Strengthening systems for the control of precursor chemicals used in the manufacture of synthetic drugs".[4] That resolution requests Governments to provide voluntarily to the Board annual estimates of their legitimate requirements for imports of the following four precursors of amphetamine-type stimulants: ephedrine, pseudoephedrine, 3,4-methylenedioxyphenyl-2-propanone (3,4-MDP-2-P) and 1-phenyl-2-propanone (P-2-P), and preparations containing those substances that could be easily used or recovered by readily applicable means.

26. Since the first publication of annual legitimate requirements in the Board's 2006 report on precursors, the number of Governments that have provided at least one estimate to the Board has doubled, and the total number of estimates substantially increased, from 160 (in 2006) to 851 (in 2016). The increase in both the number of Governments providing at least one estimate and the number of the individual estimates confirms that these estimates continue to be a useful tool for Governments to assess the legitimacy of shipments and to identify any excesses in pre-export notifications. First-time submissions of annual legitimate requirements were made by Burundi, Cabo Verde, Ethiopia, Oman and Rwanda, which brought the total number of submitting Governments to 162 as at 1 November 2016. The authorities of Ethiopia submitted estimates for ephedrine (1,000 kg) and pseudoephedrine preparations (100 kg). In 2016, more than 90 countries and territories have followed the recommendations of the Board and reconfirmed or updated the annual legitimate requirements for at least one of the four substances and their preparations, and more than half of them have reconfirmed or updated the annual legitimate requirements for all substances in question.

27. One of the most significant updates includes the reduced estimates for P-2-P and 3,4-MDP-2-P from the Government of Zimbabwe. As stated in previous reports, the Government of Zimbabwe had, for two consecutive years, submitted estimates of 1,000 litres for each of those two substances. Recently, the Government clarified this issue and the estimates were corrected to zero accordingly. INCB is also in the process of clarifying proposed upward revisions of estimates provided by the Indian authorities, in particular with regard to ephedrine and pseudoephedrine and their preparations. The Government of Afghanistan confirmed that it will not authorize any imports of pseudoephedrine raw materials into its territory.

28. Hungary has revised significantly upwards its annual legitimate requirement for the import of P-2-P, from 800 to 1,800 litres. The substance is being used in pharmaceutical production in that country. It is of note that worldwide, only 23 countries have indicated a need to import P-2-P.

29. In its 2012 and 2015 reports on precursors, INCB stated that several Governments, when establishing annual legitimate requirements for precursor chemicals, appeared to have built in "safety margins" that are far above the actual amounts required for import into the respective country. **INCB commends all Governments that have established realistic annual legitimate requirements or regularly review existing ones, thus providing the competent authorities of exporting countries with at least an indication of their needs and alerting authorities to any potential oversupply.**

30. In response to concern expressed by INCB about high estimated annual legitimate requirements for pseudoephedrine, the Government of the Syrian Arab Republic informed the Board of a series of measures taken to increase control over the substance. Those measures included import quotas for individual companies and a requirement to submit monthly reports about the use of imported quantities and the sales of any further refined products (decision 22/1452 issued on 13 July 2014). Importantly, a moratorium on the approval of pseudoephedrine imports had been imposed from late 2015 until mid-2016. The Government also confirmed the annual legitimate requirement of 50 tons, which had remained unchanged since 2007 although the number of pharmaceutical companies has increased during the same period. Finally, the Government informed the Board that as a result of the current situation in the Syrian Arab Republic, manufacturing contracts between pharmaceutical companies had been drawn up allowing companies in conflict areas, such as Aleppo, to import pseudoephedrine and process it in safer parts of the

---

[4] The latest estimates submitted by Governments are provided in annex II; regular updates are published on the Board's website.

country. INCB continues its dialogue with the Syrian authorities to ensure that remaining concerns are addressed and its dialogue with all Governments to ensure that heightened levels of vigilance are maintained, particularly towards large-scale orders of pseudoephedrine by Syrian companies, thus contributing to balancing the need to ensure adequate supplies of the substance with preventing diversion into illicit channels.

G. Pre-export notifications and utilization of the PEN Online system

31. Pre-export notifications are at the core of the system to monitor international trade in substances in Tables I and II of the 1988 Convention. In order for the pre-export notification system to be effective, Governments must formally invoke article 12, paragraph 10 (a), to make it mandatory for the authorities of exporting countries to send pre-export notifications. Although not a treaty-mandated requirement, Governments should also register with the INCB automated online system for the exchange of pre-export notifications, PEN Online, to ensure that they receive information about all relevant planned shipments of chemicals destined for their territory in real time, before those shipments leave the exporting country.

1. Pre-export notifications

32. Since the publication of the Board's 2015 report on precursors, Georgia, Myanmar and Uruguay invoked article 12, paragraph 10 (a), for all substances in Tables I and II, thus bringing the number of Governments that have formally requested to receive pre-export notifications as at 1 November 2016 to 112 (see map 1 and annex X). **INCB welcomes the invocations by the three countries but regrets that this important tool for preventing the diversion of precursors from international trade continues to be underutilized, including in some regions, such as Africa and Oceania, as well as parts of Europe.**

33. INCB wishes to remind Governments that shipments dispatched without pre-export notifications are at greater risk of being diverted, in particular those shipments destined for countries that do not have in place a control system based on individual import permits. Information on the systems of authorization that Governments apply to the import (and export) of substances in Tables I and II of the 1988 Convention is available in the Board's information package on the control of precursors, accessible to competent national authorities on the Board's secure website.

Map 1. Governments that have registered with the Pre-Export Notification Online system and those that have invoked article 12, paragraph 10 (a), of the 1988 Convention, requiring pre-export notification for selected substances (As at 1 November 2016)

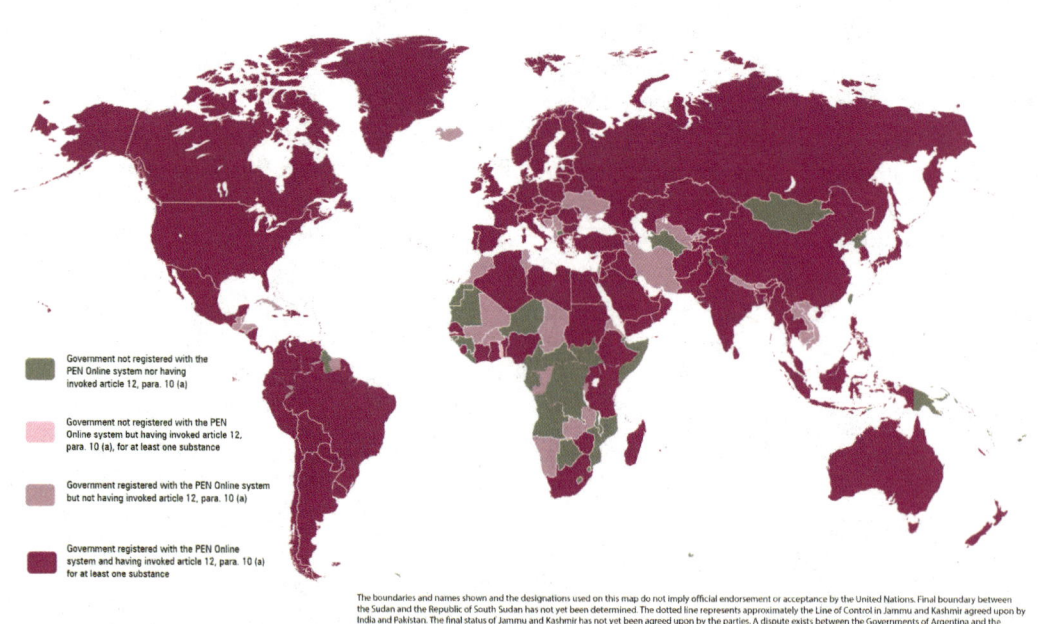

2. Pre-export Notification Online system

34. PEN Online, the automated online system for the exchange of pre-export notifications, has become the most effective tool for Governments to monitor, and communicate about matters related to, international trade in scheduled precursors worldwide and in real time.

35. With the registration of the Gambia and Tunisia, as at 1 November 2016, 153 countries and territories had access to the PEN Online system (see map 1). From among the 44 countries and territories not yet registered with PEN Online,[5] 22 are in Africa and 10 in Oceania; the authorities of major trading countries are all registered and use the system actively. INCB welcomes the registration of the Gambia and Tunisia and urges Governments that have not yet done so to register with the PEN Online system without further delay.

36. INCB would once again like to remind Governments that registration with the PEN Online system does not automatically invoke article 12, paragraph 10 (a), or vice versa. Currently, there are 50 countries and territories, including the Gambia and Tunisia, that have registered to use the PEN Online system but have not yet invoked article 12, paragraph 10 (a);[6] Antigua and Barbuda, Cayman Islands, Maldives, Togo and Tonga have invoked the article but are not registered with PEN Online (see map 1).

37. The level of active utilization of PEN Online has increased with the release of the upgraded system in October 2015. However, there are a number of registered importing Governments that do not actively utilize the system and thus remain vulnerable to the diversion of precursors. In 2015, this was the case for 22 Governments of which 11 are in Africa, 5 in Central America and the Caribbean, 4 in Europe and 2 in West Asia. INCB encourages the authorities of all importing countries, as a minimum, to review all incoming pre-export notifications and to respond to them in those cases where a response is explicitly requested by the exporting country's authorities.

38. In terms of shipments notified through the PEN Online system, about 70 per cent and 30 per cent of pre-export notifications each year involve substances in, respectively, Table II and Table I; more than 60 per cent of the notifications involve preparations containing ephedrine and pseudoephedrine, in line with Commission on Narcotic Drugs resolution 54/8. INCB commends all exporting Governments that use PEN Online actively and systematically, that is, Governments that notify the authorities of importing countries of every planned export prior to dispatching it, including exports of pharmaceutical preparations containing ephedrine or pseudoephedrine. At the same time, INCB would like to remind the authorities of exporting countries to allow sufficient time, typically between 5 and 10 working days, for the importing country's authorities to verify the legitimacy of a shipment.

39. Since 1 November 2015, nearly 30,000 pre-export notifications were sent through PEN Online; more than 2,200 shipments, or about 7.5 per cent of all pre-notified shipments, have been objected to through PEN Online by the authorities of the importing countries. A number of objections were for administrative reasons; cases of suspended and stopped shipments are included in the relevant sections of chapter III.

40. The analysis of licit trade data provided by importing countries on form D and of PEN Online data suggests that there continue to be exports of substances in Table I of the 1988 Convention without pre-export notifications through PEN Online. For the fourth consecutive year, this is the case of exports of acetic anhydride from Saudi Arabia to the Republic of Korea. In addition, Indonesia reported on form D having exported almost 50,000 litres of safrole to China but no pre-export notification was ever sent through PEN Online. INCB encourages the Government of Indonesia to register all relevant competent authorities under article 12 of the 1988 Convention to PEN Online, or to establish a working mechanism to ensure that pre-export notifications can be sent for all relevant industrial chemicals under international control as well.

41. The Board's last report on precursors referred to information provided by the authorities of Pakistan on form D

---

[5] Angola, Antigua and Barbuda, Botswana, Cameroon, Central African Republic, Comoros, Democratic People's Republic of Korea, Democratic Republic of the Congo, Djibouti, Dominica, Equatorial Guinea, Fiji, Gabon, Guinea, Guinea-Bissau, Guyana, Kiribati, Kuwait, Lesotho, Liberia, Malawi, Maldives, Mauritania, Monaco, Mongolia, Mozambique, Nauru, Niger, Palau, Papua New Guinea, Saint Kitts and Nevis, Samoa, San Marino, Sao Tome and Principe, Somalia, South Sudan, Swaziland, the former Yugoslav Republic of Macedonia, Timor-Leste, Togo, Tonga, Turkmenistan, Tuvalu and Vanuatu.

[6] Albania, Andorra, Bahamas, Bahrain, Belize, Bhutan, Bosnia and Herzegovina, Brunei Darussalam, Burkina Faso, Burundi, Cabo Verde, Cambodia, Chad, Congo, Cuba, Eritrea, Gambia, Georgia, Grenada, Guatemala, Honduras, Iceland, Iran (Islamic Republic of), Israel, Lao People's Democratic Republic, Mali, Marshall Islands, Mauritius, Micronesia (Federated States of), Montenegro, Morocco, Myanmar, Namibia, Nepal, New Zealand, Rwanda, Saint Lucia, Senegal, Serbia, Seychelles, Solomon Islands, Suriname, Tunisia, Uganda, Ukraine, Uruguay, Uzbekistan, Viet Nam, Yemen and Zambia.

for 2014 about imports of phenylacetic acid from China and India. The Pakistani authorities have since then clarified that there were no imports of phenylacetic acid during 2014.

H. Activities and achievements in international precursor control

1. Project Prism and Project Cohesion

42. The two international initiatives led by INCB, Project Prism and Project Cohesion, continue to serve as platforms for international cooperation in matters related to chemicals used in the illicit manufacture of, respectively, amphetamine-type stimulants, and heroin and cocaine. As at 1 November 2016, 134 and 92 countries had nominated focal points for activities under Project Prism and Project Cohesion, respectively. International and regional bodies such as the European Commission, the International Criminal Police Organization (INTERPOL), the Inter-American Drug Abuse Control Commission of the Organization of American States, the United Nations Office on Drugs and Crime (UNODC) and the World Customs Organization also participate in the two projects. Both projects are steered by the INCB Precursors Task Force, which met twice in 2016, inter alia, to coordinate a global survey to identify the sources and modi operandi to obtain fentanyl, fentanyl analogues, other opioid-type new psychoactive substances, and the related precursors, as well as an international operation focusing on international trade in and smuggling of amphetamine and methamphetamine precursors, including chemicals used in the illicit manufacture of the drugs presumed to be present in "captagon" tablets currently trafficked.[7] The results of the survey and the operation, which is known as Operation Missing Links, will be evaluated by the Task Force in an upcoming meeting and disseminated to participating Governments. INCB thanks those Governments that actively participated in the activities and encourages them to continue to provide information about substances that could be used in the illicit manufacture of fentanyls and the drugs found in "captagon" tablets currently trafficked as well as about the modi operandi of traffickers, to allow for a comprehensive analysis of this issue and devise adequate measures to address it.

---

[7] The term "captagon" is used to refer to what is available today in the illicit markets in countries in the Middle East. The composition of the product has nothing in common with "Captagon", the pharmaceutical product that was available starting in the early 1960s and which contained the substance fenethylline.

43. PICS enables ongoing, real-time communication among participants in the two projects (see below). Participants in Project Prism and Project Cohesion are also informed, by means of special alerts, about major precursor trafficking trends, modi operandi of diversions and attempted diversions and newly emerging precursors. Since the last report on precursors, eight alerts were issued that informed Project Prism and Project Cohesion focal points about attempted diversions of ergot alkaloids involving companies in Suriname; a number of non-scheduled chemicals, including a precursor of mephedrone and a substitute chemical for APAAN; the modi operandi for the smuggling of non-scheduled synthetic drug precursors in buckets and for the smuggling of acetic anhydride disguised as glacial acetic acid; and information gaps in relation to the sources of precursors used in illicit methamphetamine manufacture in the Golden Triangle. One alert also provided the results of Operation MMA, a global operation which targeted methylamine (monomethylamine), a chemical not under international control that is required in the illicit manufacture of a number of drugs (such as methamphetamine and 3,4-methylenedioxymethamphetamine (MDMA)), the precursor ephedrine and several new psychoactive substances (especially synthetic cathinones).

44. The Precursors Task Force has in recent years repeatedly encouraged international operational cooperation in relation to chemicals used in the illicit processing of cocaine and heroin. However, there has been little interest, including in the regions most affected, in a global, targeted activity to shed light on the sources of those required chemicals and their substitutes. INCB encourages all Governments to make use of the existing global cooperation mechanisms under Project Prism and Project Cohesion to gather and exchange information on new trafficking trends, on modi operandi and on the criminal organizations involved and how they operate, and to use that knowledge to develop specific risk profiles and conduct joint operations to prevent future diversions. INCB also reiterates its recommendations to all Governments to ensure that the contact details of their focal points for Project Prism and Project Cohesion are always up-to-date and that those focal points actively participate in the relevant operations under Project Prism and Project Cohesion and follow-up on the action identified.

2. Precursors Incident Communication System

45. Since its launch in March 2012, PICS has become an important component of the toolbox for global operational cooperation in precursor matters. The communication platform allows Government authorities to share information

in real time about individual precursor incidents such as seizures, shipments stopped in transit and illicit laboratories, involving scheduled and non-scheduled substances. The early communication of such information alerts users to emerging trends in chemicals and, specifically, alerts the authorities of the countries involved in an incident, as a source, transit or destination country, or when a national of that country is involved, and allows the users to contact each other for further details and to launch joint investigations.[8]

46. Utilization of PICS, which is available in English, French, Russian and Spanish, is cost-free. Since the publication of the last report on precursors, 59 users from 41 agencies in 26 countries have newly registered to use PICS (see map 2),[9] bringing the number of users to nearly 450, agencies to 214 and countries to 100. With the 212 incidents communicated since 1 November 2015, the total number of incidents communicated through PICS has reached almost 1,700, involving more than 90 different countries and territories; 30 per cent of those incidents involved chemicals not under international control, including substances on the limited international special surveillance list. An increasing proportion of incidents now also have actionable information, such as routing information (source, transit and destination), company information, relevant documentation and the names used to disguise the identity of the chemicals, which provide a solid starting point for investigations in the countries concerned. INCB commends all PICS users that share information on individual precursor incidents with sufficient operational detail to allow the users of other countries involved in an incident to initiate requisite follow-up investigations with a view to not only bring to justice those behind the specific incident in question but also to deny traffickers access to chemicals using similar modi operandi in the future.

Map 2. Governments registered with and that are using the Precursors Incident Communication System
(As at 1 November 2016)

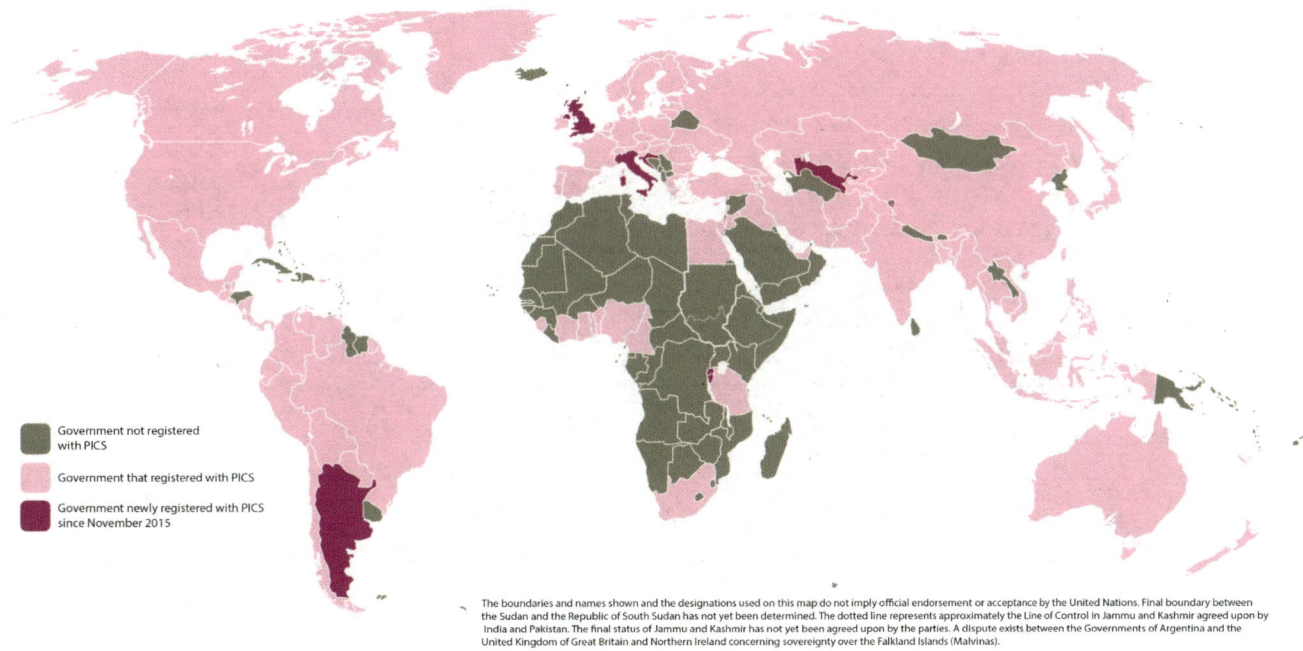

---

[8] For further details about PICS and the minimum action for sharing information about precursor incidents through the system, see box 3 in the INCB report on precursors for 2015 (E/INCB/2015/4).

[9] Governments that have not yet registered PICS focal points for their relevant national authorities involved in precursor control may request an account at the following e-mail address: pics@incb.org.

III. Extent of licit trade in precursors and the latest trends in precursor trafficking

47. The following analysis provides an overview of the major trends and developments identified for both the licit trade in precursor chemicals and the trafficking in these substances. The analysis is based on data provided by

Governments on form D for 2015. Other sources of information include PEN Online, Project Prism and Project Cohesion, PICS and direct notifications from Governments including national reports. That information was drawn on to identify developments for the period 1 November 2015 to 1 November 2016. INCB wishes to thank Governments for the information received, in particular those Governments that provided information on specific cases of diversion, trafficking and activities associated with illicit drug manufacture.

48. With regard to data on seizures, readers should bear in mind that reported seizures generally reflect the corresponding level of regulatory and law enforcement activity at that specific time. In addition, as seizures are often the result of law enforcement cooperation among several countries (e.g., through controlled deliveries), the occurrence and magnitude of seizures made in a given country should not be misinterpreted or overestimated in assessing that country's role in the overall situation of trafficking in precursors. From the point of view of precursor control, that is, with a view to addressing gaps and weaknesses in control mechanisms, the amounts seized are of secondary importance; rather, it is the information and intelligence generated from a seizure, a stopped or suspended shipment, theft, attempted diversion or a suspicious order or even inquiry, that is critical for preventing future diversions of chemicals. INCB therefore encourages all Governments to improve the quality and comprehensiveness of their annual form D submissions and to make better use of PICS.

49. Given the widespread legitimate uses of a number of the substances in Tables I and II of the 1988 Convention, there is significant international trade in most precursors used in the illicit manufacture of drugs. Between 1 November 2015 and 1 November 2016, the authorities of 67 exporting countries used the PEN Online system for almost 30,000 transactions. Volumes of trade and the number of shipments vary significantly depending on the substance and from one year to another.

A. Substances used in the illicit manufacture of amphetamine-type stimulants

50. Pre-export notifications involving precursors of amphetamine-type stimulants account for about 65 per cent of all pre-export notifications for Table I substances sent between 1 November 2015 and 1 November 2016: the authorities of 42 exporting countries used the PEN Online system for almost 5,600 transactions involving shipments of precursors of amphetamine-type stimulants. Likewise, precursors of amphetamine-type stimulants represent 43 per cent of incidents communicated through PICS. Those numbers are comparable to those for the previous year.

1. Substances used in the illicit manufacture of amphetamines

(a) Ephdrine and pseudoephedrine

51. Ephedrine and pseudoephedrine are among the most widely used precursors for the illicit manufacture of methamphetamine. They are also both used legitimately for medical purposes and are therefore among the most frequently and widely traded substances in Table I of the 1988 Convention, both in the form of raw materials as well as pharmaceutical preparations. P-2-P, phenylacetic acid and APAAN, as well as a number of non-scheduled substances, may be used to substitute for, or as alternatives to, ephedrine and pseudoephedrine in illicit methamphetamine manufacture (see paras. 98-110 and annex IV).

Licit trade

52. Details regarding 4,912 notifications of planned shipments of ephedrine and pseudoephedrine, in bulk (raw material) and in the form of pharmaceutical preparations, were submitted through the PEN Online system between 1 November 2015 and 1 November 2016. The shipments consisted of a total of 952 tons of pseudoephedrine and 104 tons of ephedrine. The shipments originated in 39 exporting countries and territories and were destined for 166 importing countries and territories. The largest exporters by volume were India and Germany, and the largest importers were the United States and the Republic of Korea.

53. In the reporting period, shipments of ephedrine and pseudoephedrine were stopped at the request of both importing and exporting countries. Canada, Hungary, India and Madagascar reported stopped shipments of ephedrine and pseudoephedrine on form D for 2015, often for administrative reasons. Through the PEN Online system, the authorities of a number of additional importing countries objected to planned shipments, again, mostly for administrative reasons. Among exporting countries, the authorities of India reported on form D having stopped shipments of 200 kg of ephedrine and 25 kg of pseudoephedrine at the request of the importing countries' competent authority through PEN Online.

54. No thefts of ephedrines were reported on form D for 2015. In 2016, two cases of thefts of pseudoephedrine, involving a total of 350 kg from shipments amounting to 3.5 tons, were brought to the attention of INCB. Both cases

involved shipments from India, one destined for Turkey and one for Egypt. INCB has followed up with all countries concerned; investigations are ongoing. INCB encourages all Governments to cooperate with each other and thoroughly investigate thefts of precursor consignments, or parts thereof, and share relevant findings, especially about the modi operandi, with INCB for further dissemination. The information will help to improve understanding of recent patterns and methods of diversion of precursor chemicals and will assist INCB and competent national authorities in preventing future diversions.

Trafficking

55. In 2015, 29 countries and territories reported on form D seizures of ephedrine either as raw material or in the form of pharmaceutical preparations. Total seizures of ephedrine raw material amounted to more than 25 tons, with China alone accounting for almost 23.5 tons, followed by New Zealand with more than 950 kg, Australia (457 kg), India (97 kg) and Malaysia (75 kg). With slightly more than 220 kg, China also reported the largest seizures of preparations containing ephedrine.

56. Pseudoephedrine seizures were reported by 24 countries and territories. However, with the exception of India (730 kg) and the United States (210 kg), none of the amounts reported by individual countries exceeded 100 kg, neither as raw material nor in the form of pharmaceutical preparations. While there had been significant fluctuation until 2013, since then the statistics on the reported seizures of the different types of ephedrines reveal an increasing predominance of seizures of ephedrine raw material (see figure II).

Figure II. Seizures of ephedrine and pseudoephedrine reported by Governments on form D, 2011-2015

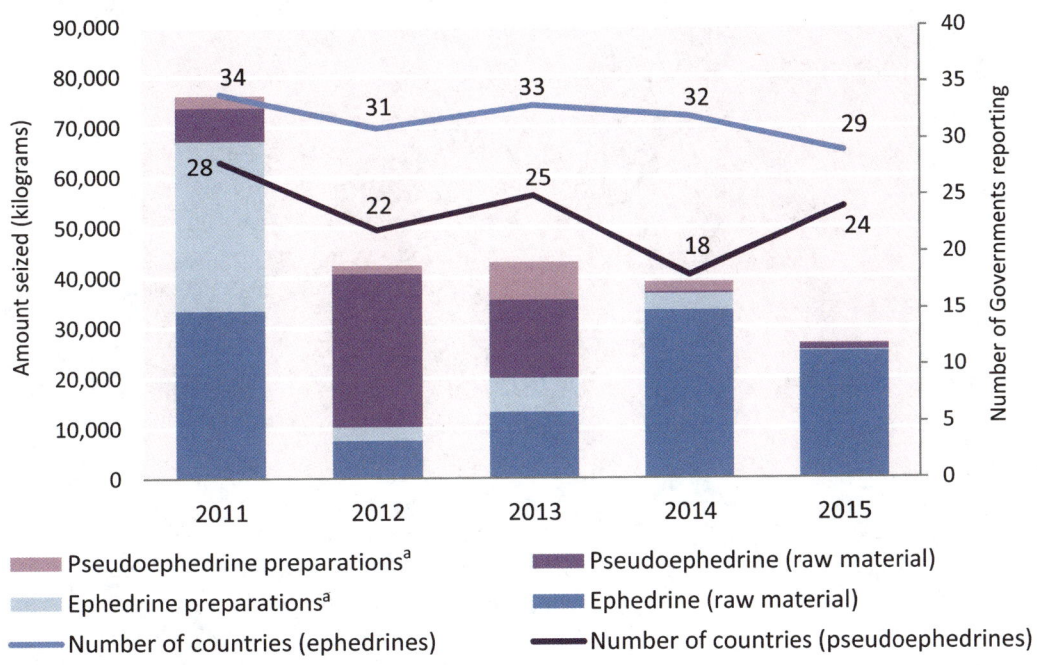

[a] Excludes preparations reported as tablets.

57. Countries in West Asia have traditionally reported few seizures of ephedrines, typically in amounts of less than 50 kg per country and year. An exception was the Islamic Republic of Iran in 2010 and 2011, when more than 6.5 tons of ephedrine raw material were seized. In Pakistan, in that same two-year period 2010-2011, slightly more than 550 kg were seized. Since then, the amounts seized in the region have been negligible, and in 2015, no ephedrine or pseudoephedrine seizures were reported by any country in West Asia.

58. According to the annual reports on drug control in the Islamic Republic of Iran, in 2015, for the third consecutive year, there was a decreasing trend in the number of dismantled laboratories, presumably mostly methamphetamine laboratories (see figure III).[10] At the same time, INCB is aware that authorities in Afghanistan are increasingly concerned about methamphetamine trafficking, abuse and illicit manufacture in their territory. Anecdotal information suggests that pharmaceutical preparations containing ephedrine and pseudoephedrine may feed some of the illicit

---

[10] Islamic Republic of Iran, Drug Control Headquarters, *Drug Control in 2015* (Tehran, March 2016); and previous years' reports.

methamphetamine manufacture, an observation that has led the Afghan authorities to control the import and export of such products. According to those authorities, illicit methamphetamine manufacture in Afghanistan occurs mostly in the provinces along the Afghan-Iranian border, often in areas outside government control; much of the methamphetamine is smuggled to the Islamic Republic of Iran.

Figure III. Number of laboratories dismantled in the Islamic Republic of Iran, 2008-2015

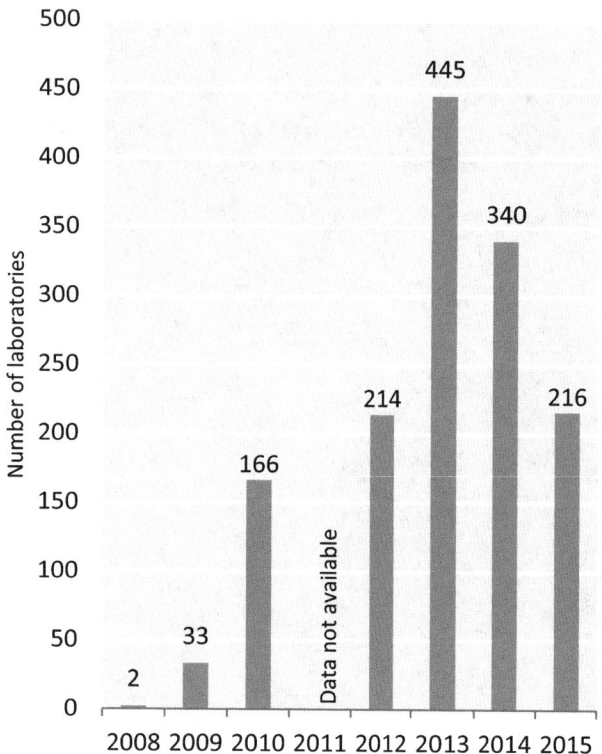

59. INCB continues to be concerned about the unclear situation with regard to trafficking in ephedrine and pseudoephedrine and their substitute or alternate precursors in other parts of West Asia, especially in countries in or neighbouring conflict areas, and with respect to the illicit manufacture of fake "captagon" tablets (see above). While illicit laboratories compressing amphetamine powder and other ingredients into "captagon" tablets are occasionally reported, there are very few reports of illicit laboratories synthesizing amphetamine or reports of seizures of the chemicals needed in such syntheses (see also para. 83, below).

60. In East and South-East Asia, significant seizures of ephedrines have been reported over the years by Myanmar (more than 3.2 tons of pseudoephedrine and 1.6 tons of ephedrine preparations in 2009, and nearly 3.6 tons of pseudoephedrine preparations in 2013), the Lao People's Democratic Republic (more than 4.6 tons of pseudoephedrine preparations in 2009), Malaysia (about 900 kg of pseudoephedrine in 2011) and the Philippines (more than 600 kg of pseudoephedrine in 2013). However, over the years, the most significant amounts have been reported by the authorities of China. In 2015, that country accounted for more than 99 per cent of all ephedrine seizures reported on form D by countries in East and South-East Asia. Although detailed information is not available, it appears that at least part of the ephedrine recently seized in China was illicitly manufactured from 2-bromopropiophenone, a precursor of ephedrine that is not under international control but has been scheduled in China since May 2014.

61. Seizures of ephedrines reported by countries other than China in East and South-East Asia in 2015 rarely exceeded 50 kg, including a few countries that had reported larger amounts in the past, such as Malaysia, Myanmar and the Philippines. Illicit methamphetamine laboratory incidents were reported by only Japan, Malaysia and the Philippines. The low number and limited amounts of seizures of ephedrine and pseudoephedrine contrast sharply with seizure data for methamphetamine end-product (both crystalline methamphetamine and methamphetamine tablets) for which there is a large and growing market in East and South-East Asia.[11] Those low numbers and amounts also contrast with other indicators that have long pointed to the Mekong river subregion as a source of illicit methamphetamine, in particular methamphetamine tablets. For example, information available from China for the years 2013-2015 suggests that while most of the crystalline methamphetamine ("ice") seized in the country is manufactured domestically, the majority of methamphetamine tablets seized in China originated in northern Myanmar.[12] At the same time, and with the exception of China, there have been very few reports in recent years of seizures of other methamphetamine precursors, or non-scheduled substitutes, in countries in East and South-East Asia.

62. China also has long been a source of ephedrines seized in countries in Oceania, namely Australia and New Zealand. Gradually tightened controls in China since 2012 and bilateral cooperation agreements between those countries and China appear to have improved the situation with regard to the specific product, which has long dominated seizures in Australia and New Zealand, i.e., pseudoephedrine

---

[11] *World Drug Report 2016* (United Nations publication, Sales No. E.16.XI.7), p. 53.

[12] National Narcotics Control Commission of China, *Annual Report on Drug Control in China 2013* (Beijing, 2013) and *Annual Report on Drug Control in China 2015* (Beijing, 2015).

preparations in the form of "ContacNT". Starting around 2014, both countries reported a significant drop in pseudoephedrine seizures, reflected also in fewer detections of illicit laboratories extracting pseudoephedrine.[13] Since then, seizures of so-called "ContacNT" have largely been replaced by seizures of ephedrine, which accounted for 95 per cent of border seizures in New Zealand in the period 2014-2015. Cooperation between the authorities of China and New Zealand resulted in the seizure of 88 kg of ephedrine in New Zealand in 2015.[14]

63. In the first eight months of 2016, the frequency of ephedrine seizures at New Zealand's borders had decreased to about half the rate of seizures in 2015. However, the quantities involved in the individual seizures increased. Although ephedrine is the most seized precursor at the border, pseudoephedrine is still the main precursor found in clandestine laboratories in New Zealand, most of which are relatively small in scale, often mobile or on private premises. In 2015, 45 laboratories were dismantled.

64. In Australia, seizures of pseudoephedrine raw materials in 2015 amounted to slightly more than 72 kg, in nearly 260 incidents. The largest single amount seized (almost 10.5 kg) was traced to Kenya, while the origin of the vast majority of seizures was unknown.

65. The authorities in Kenya also reported seizures of ephedrine (18.2 kg) in 2015, for the first time in five years, and the country is alleged to be the destination of smuggled ephedrine from India (see para. 69, below). INCB is also aware of a seizure of 12.5 kg of ephedrine in Mali, arriving from Guinea, and a seizure of nearly 280 kg of ephedrine in Côte d'Ivoire, presumably for use as such, as a mild stimulant. The use of ephedrine to cut cocaine has also been reported by authorities in Africa.

66. South Africa continued to be a destination for the smuggling of significant amounts of methamphetamine precursors in 2016. A single seizure in June 2016 involved 140 kg of ephedrine. In May 2016, South African police dismantled an illicit methamphetamine laboratory and seized 12 kg of the drug, as well as a variety of chemicals and drug manufacturing equipment; investigations are ongoing. **INCB regrets that South Africa has effectively stopped providing mandatory seizure information on precursors in 2008, and regrets that the Board has not been able to confirm seizure information available on official government websites. INCB encourages the South African authorities to fulfil their international obligations and their role as an important partner in countering illicit drug manufacture and precursor trafficking.**

67. In Africa, illicit methamphetamine manufacture was also reported by the authorities in Nigeria. While between 2013 and 2015, 10 laboratories illicitly manufacturing methamphetamine from ephedrines had been found in Nigeria, it was in March 2016 that the Nigerian authorities, for the first time, dismantled an industrial-scale laboratory. Worryingly, not only did the laboratory significantly exceed the scale of previously detected laboratories but also the manufacturing method it used was based on chemicals not under international control (see para. 101, below).

68. Seizures of ephedrines in South Asia have been reported almost exclusively by India. Ephedrine seizures in that country peaked in 2011 and pseudoephedrine seizures peaked in 2012 and 2013. The sharp decline after 2013 (see figure IV) is attributable, according to the Indian authorities, to the strengthening of domestic controls, namely the mandatory registration of operators involved in the manufacture, distribution, sale, purchase, possession, storage or consumption of substances in schedule-A of the Narcotic Drugs and Psychotropic Substances (Regulation of Controlled Substances) Order.[15] India has also occasionally reported illicit manufacture of ephedrine. One such illicit facility was dismantled in July 2016, and 45 kg of ephedrine seized.

69. In April 2016, Indian authorities seized in a single incident more than 10 tons of ephedrine and 8.5 tons of pseudoephedrine, amounts that exceeded by far the total seizures in any one year in the past; the substances were seized from the warehouse of a pharmaceutical company. While INCB understands that investigations are ongoing, there have been claims that the company had been targeted since 2013 and that the ephedrine was intended to be smuggled to Kenya and the United Republic of Tanzania for illicit methamphetamine manufacture, involving international trafficking networks. It is claimed that the case highlights the shortage of drug inspectors for regular inspections at manufacturing and selling units, as well as the dangers of small, financially distressed companies being targeted by traffickers. According to the media, the last inspection of the company was in July 2015, when no violations were observed. However, since the substances had allegedly been stocked for several years as a by-product of the ephedrine manufacturing process, the inspectors did not know the stock existed. The most recent media reports suggested that in addition to the ephedrine by-product having been smuggled outside India,

---

[13] Australian Criminal Intelligence Commission, *Illicit Drug Data Report 2014-2015*, p. 155.

[14] China, National Narcotics Control Commission, *Annual Report on Drug Control in China 2016* (Beijing, 2016).

[15] India, Ministry of Home Affairs, *Annual Report 2015* (New Delhi, Narcotics Control Bureau, 2015), p. 27.

the company had also been used to manufacture ephedrine specifically to be smuggled abroad. INCB commends Governments for uncovering diversion attempts and effecting precursor seizures. However, INCB would like to remind Governments of the importance of thoroughly investigating all diversion attempts and seizures, and communicating relevant findings to INCB and any other countries concerned so that the underlying weaknesses of domestic monitoring systems or shortcomings at the international level can be addressed.

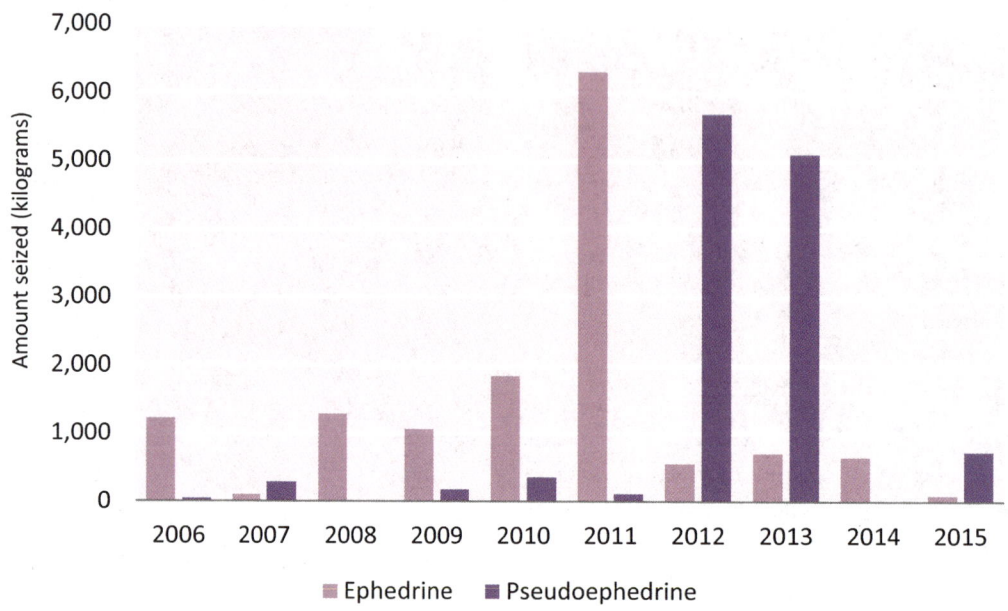

Figure IV. Seizures of ephedrine and pseudoephedrine raw materials reported on form D by the Government of India, 2006-2015

Note: Excludes seizures of preparations containing ephedrine or pseudoephedrine, which were typically reported as tablets. In 2014, India reported having seized 676 kg of pseudoephedrine preparations.

70. In a similar case, in July 2016, authorities in Nepal seized nearly 500 kg of pseudoephedrine from the premises of a company in Kathmandu. While investigations are ongoing, INCB understands that the substance was legitimately imported, then manufactured into preparations containing pseudoephedrine, which were subsequently seized from the premises of a packaging company; the substance was to be smuggled abroad. **While commending the Nepalese authorities for the seizure, INCB encourages the authorities to review the annual legitimate requirements for imports of pseudoephedrine into Nepal (currently 5,000 kg) and amend them on the basis of the most recent market data. INCB encourages all other countries to regularly review and update, as required, the annual legitimate requirements for imports of a number of amphetamine-type stimulant precursors as well.**

71. In Europe in 2015, seizures of ephedrines mostly involved preparations containing pseudoephedrine. That is similar to the situation in 2014, although the amounts reported in 2015 were significantly smaller, totalling just about 225 kg. In 2015, the largest amounts were reported by Czechia (nearly 77 kg, in 120 incidents) and Bulgaria (nearly 66 kg), followed by Ukraine (47 kg) and Poland (35 kg). Bulgaria also reported seizures of pseudoephedrine raw material, while seizures of ephedrine both as raw material and in the form of preparations were negligible in Europe — the largest seizure involved about 4 kg of ephedrine in a postal air shipment from India to Germany.

72. Tablets containing pseudoephedrine seized in Czechia typically contained more than 30 mg (and up to 120 mg) of pseudoephedrine per dosage unit and were destined for one of the 262 small-scale illicit methamphetamine laboratories dismantled in 2015. Turkey continued to be identified as a country of origin. Seizures of preparations containing pseudoephedrine also continued in 2016, as communicated through PICS, although a decrease in the number of such incidents suggests that the measures taken by the authorities in Turkey are having some effect. **INCB reminds Governments to consider, to the extent possible and in accordance with national legislation, applying control measures for pharmaceutical preparations containing ephedrine or pseudoephedrine similar to those for the bulk (raw) substances.**

73. Among all countries having reported seizures of ephedrines, the United States recorded the largest decrease in a five-year period. In 2015, the country reported only a seizure of slightly more than 210 kg involving 37,200 bottles of various pseudoephedrine-antihistamine combination preparations. Investigations determined that the bottles were stolen in 2010, when they were placed on a trailer from a business that the local pharmacy board had shut down, and the owner of the business was supposed to pay to have the products destroyed, but they were then reported stolen. A number of the bottles appeared at a police traffic stop in June 2015 and resulted in the recovery of the trailer with the remainder of the bottles.

74. Even with high-purity methamphetamine being smuggled into the United States, illicit manufacture of the drug has continued in the country. As in the past, and although it continues to decrease, such small-scale domestic manufacture is fuelled by pharmaceutical products containing ephedrine and pseudoephedrine, obtained through a series of purchases from multiple retail outlets to circumvent established purchase limits (known as "smurfing"), and the use of crude manufacturing methods such as the "one-pot method".

75. In the rest of North America, Mexico did not report any seizures of ephedrines on form D for 2015, while Canada reported negligible amounts. The situation was similar in Central and South America and the Caribbean, where only Argentina reported a notable seizure of ephedrine on form D for 2015, of an amount of less than 50 kg.

(b) Norephedrine and ephedra

Licit trade

76. International trade in norephedrine, a substance which can be used in the illicit manufacture of amphetamine, continues to be low compared with trade in other precursors of amphetamine-type stimulants. Between 1 November 2015 and 1 November 2016, 174 transactions involving norephedrine were recorded through the PEN Online system: 12 exporting countries pre-notified shipments to 28 importing countries, amounting to more than 33 tons of raw material and 19.5 tons in the form of pharmaceutical preparations. Shipments amounting to 1 ton or more were pre-notified to the following importing countries, in descending order: United States, India, Myanmar, Algeria, Cambodia, Phillippines and Sweden.

Trafficking

77. Seizures of norephedrine were reported on form D for 2015 by only four countries: Australia, China, Philippines and Ukraine; the amounts were all less than 15 kg, seized in multiple incidents, i.e., individual seizures were small and the origins mostly unknown. There were no seizures of ephedra reported on form D. However, according to information in its annual report, China seized 146 tons of ephedra in 2015, the lowest amount in three years.[16]

(c) 1-Phenyl-2-propanone, phenylacetic acid and APAAN

78. P-2-P, phenylacetic acid and APAAN can be used in the illicit manufacture of amphetamine and methamphetamine. While P-2-P is an immediate precursor to the two drugs, it can itself be synthesized from phenylacetic acid and APAAN. Legitimate trade in the three substances differs significantly in volume, extent and the number of countries involved. Seizures of diverted P-2-P have been rare in recent years and typically involved P-2-P that was illicitly manufactured. Non-scheduled substitutes for, or alternatives to, P-2-P in the illicit manufacture of amphetamine and methamphetamine are addressed in paragraphs 98-110, below.

Licit trade

79. With very few legitimate uses other than for the manufacture of amphetamine or methamphetamine for pharmaceutical purposes, international trade in P-2-P is also very limited. Between 1 November 2015 and 1 November 2016, there were only 18 pre-export notifications for planned exports of P-2-P, from four exporting countries to 11 importing countries; the largest exporter was India and the largest importer was the United States. By contrast, licit international trade in phenylacetic acid is by far more significant and widespread, with 13 exporting countries having notified 47 importing countries and territories about 570 planned shipments of phenylacetic acid. There were no transactions involving APAAN.

80. Following an attempted import of more than 9,000 litres of P-2-P into the Syrian Arab Republic by a previously unknown company in 2014, the same company attempted to import 24 tons of phenylacetic acid in March 2016. The shipment was suspended by the Indian authorities in close coordination with INCB; investigations are ongoing. INCB welcomes the vigilance and close cooperation of Governments to prevent chemical diversion and encourages the timely exchange of all relevant documentation to enable the authorities of the countries concerned to investigate suspicious cases, diversions and attempted diversions. INCB wishes to acknowledge

---

[16] National Narcotics Control Commission of China, *Annual Report on Drug Control in China 2016*.

specifically the efforts made by the authorities of countries participating in Operation Missing Links to assist the authorities in countries where conflicts and political instability affect the ability of those authorities to effectively control the trade in precursors in their entire territory.

Trafficking

81. Seizures of P-2-P in 2015 were reported by 10 countries and territories. The largest amounts were seized by Mexico (more than 16,500 litres), Poland (nearly 7,000 litres) and China (nearly 5,500 litres), followed by the Netherlands (525 litres) and Belgium (435 litres). Other seizures were made mostly by European countries, including Estonia, Finland, Germany and Hungary and did not exceed 20 litres. Most of the P-2-P seized in 2015 was reported to have been seized in illicit laboratories where it had been illicitly manufactured from various pre-precursors (see also paras. 98-110, below); this included the total amount reported by Mexico. The seizure in Poland was the result of meticulous law enforcement investigations that are still ongoing to identify details of the methods of diversion and the trafficking organizations involved. While the integrity of ongoing investigations must be ensured, INCB encourages the authorities in the countries concerned, as well as relevant European institutions, to ensure that the details of the investigation are made available to those that need to know in order to prevent similar diversions from happening in the future and elsewhere.

82. Seven countries and territories reported seizures of phenylacetic acid on form D for 2015. The largest amounts seized — more than 16 tons — were reported by the authorities of Lebanon, followed by Mexico (550 kg) and the Netherlands (nearly 260 kg). The amounts seized in Australia, China, Spain and Ukraine did not exceed 25 kg in any country. Information about the origin or modi operandi of the traffickers was usually not provided.

83. The seizure of phenylacetic acid in Lebanon is one of the few seizures in West Asia of precursors of amphetamine, which is typically the main active ingredient in fake "captagon" tablets.[17] Lebanese authorities also confirmed the dismantling of a laboratory in Dar El Wasiaa village in December 2015 and the seizure of chemicals and equipment, which seemed to suggest that some chemical synthesis may have taken place in that laboratory. In 2016, during the pre-operational phase of Operation Missing Links, INCB also became aware of a seizure in Lebanon of about 1 ton of a solid chemical suspected of being a precursor used for manufacturing "captagon". While investigations are ongoing, INCB wishes to commend the Lebanese authorities for those seizures. INCB also wishes to encourage all Governments to be vigilant with respect to shipments of amphetamine precursors under international control, as well as non-scheduled chemicals, to countries in West Asia, as a contribution to establishing the missing links, which would help for understanding and addressing the sources of chemicals that feed the illicit production of "captagon".

84. Seizures of APAAN were reported on form D by five countries, totalling slightly more than 1.5 tons. That is a significant decrease from previous years (see figure V), especially when compared with the seizures communicated through PICS.

85. Germany reported two seizures of APAAN, totalling 37.5 kg, which originated in China and the Netherlands. In the incident involving APAAN that originated in the Netherlands, the substance was passed off as amphetamine. The larger seizure of APAAN, 35.5 kg, was identified in a mixture with 2-phenylacetoacetamide (APAA), a substance not under international control that is manufactured from, or via, APAAN, is an immediate precursor of P-2-P, and has been encountered in increasing frequency and amounts over the past year (see para. 108, below); it was seized when it was transiting Germany from China to Poland.

86. In 2016, seizures of P-2-P and APAAN continued to be communicated through PICS. In the first 10 months of 2016, eight incidents involving P-2-P, amounting to slightly less than 60 litres, and six incidents involving APAAN amounting to slightly more than 500 kg were communicated through PICS. While the majority of incidents involving both substances occurred in illicit laboratories or warehouses, often in the Netherlands, there were also incidents at airports (France), inland roads (Netherlands) and at a courier company (Mexico).

87. The example of APAAN illustrates the value of the early sharing of information through PICS and the immediate impact of controls: the voluntary communication of individual incidents through PICS contributed to building a case for the international control of APAAN in 2014. Subsequent sharing of information through PICS then revealed the dramatic decline in seizures after controls came into effect. In addition, it should be noted that reporting on form D started only after those controls were in place.

---

[17] While illicit laboratories compressing amphetamine powder and other ingredients into "captagon" tablets have occasionally been reported, there are few reports in West Asia of illicit laboratories synthesizing amphetamine or reports of seizures of the chemicals needed for such syntheses.

CHAPTER III. EXTENT OF LICIT TRADE IN PRECURSORS AND THE LATEST TRENDS IN PRECURSOR TRAFFICKING

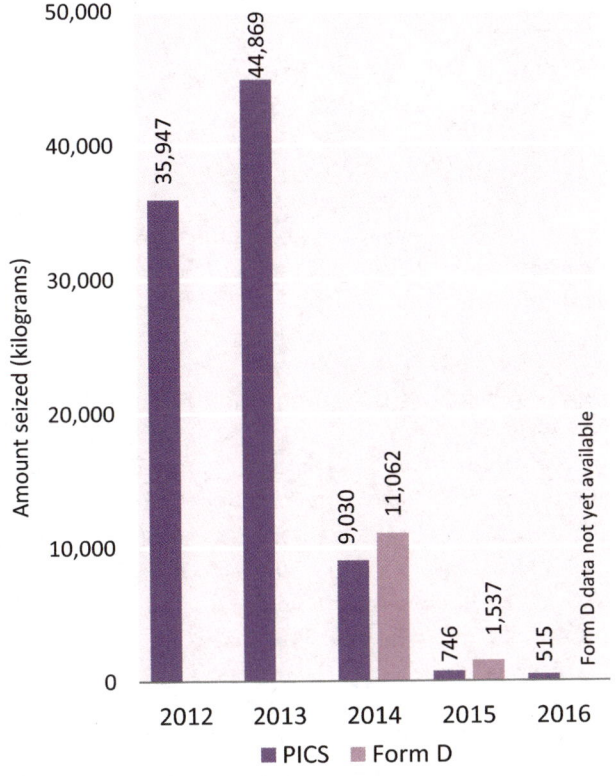

Figure V. Seizures of APAAN communicated through PICS and reported on form D, 2012-2016

Note: Reporting on form D (2012-2015).

2. Substances used in the illicit manufacture of 3,4-methylenedioxymethamphetamine and its analogues

88. 3,4-MDP-2-P is an immediate precursor to 3,4-methylenedioxymethamphetamine (MDMA) and other "ecstasy"-type substances and can itself be manufactured from piperonal, safrole or isosafrole (see annex IV). Legitimate trade in the four chemicals differs significantly in terms of volume, extent and the number of countries involved. Of the four chemicals, piperonal is the most widely traded precursor, while international trade in 3,4-MDP-2-P and isosafrole is nearly non-existent. None of the chemicals have been frequently diverted into illicit markets in recent years, perhaps with the exception of safrole and safrole-rich oils. Instead, seizures of 3,4-MDP-2-P typically involved cases in which the substance had been illicitly manufactured from non-scheduled pre-precursors (see also paras. 111-117, below).

(a) 3,4-Methylenedioxyphenyl-2-propanone and piperonal

Licit trade

89. Between 1 November 2015 and 1 November 2016, 18 exporting countries notified the authorities of 47 importing countries of 540 planned exports of piperonal, amounting to a total of nearly 1,940 tons. As in previous years, there were no pre-export notifications for 3,4-MDP-2-P.

Trafficking

90. Sizeable seizures of 3,4-MDP-2-P were reported on form D for 2015 only by the Netherlands, Australia and India, amounting to about 500 litres, 140 litres and 43 litres, respectively. One incident in Australia, involving about 90 litres, could be traced to China, while the origin of the substance seized in two further incidents is unknown. Australia and the Netherlands were also the only countries reporting seizures of piperonal in amounts greater than 1 kg. The Netherlands reported three seizures of a total of nearly 45 kg of piperonal, which were all made in illicit laboratories and warehouses. Seizures in Australia amounted to about 5.7 kg, including a mixture of 3,4-MDP-2-P and piperonal.

91. Through PICS, INCB is also aware of additional seizures of both substances in 2016. Of note is a seizure of 125 litres of 3,4-MDP-2-P, together with 375 litres of methylamine, in a warehouse in the Netherlands. Other, significantly larger seizures of non-scheduled 3,4-MDP-2-P derivatives were also communicated through PICS (see paras. 111-117, below). There were no incidents involving piperonal communicated through PICS in 2016.

(b) Safrole, safrole-rich oils and isosafrole

Licit trade

92. During the reporting period, six exporting countries sent 26 pre-export notifications for safrole and safrole-rich oils via PEN Online to 11 importing countries, involving a total volume of 2,300 litres. That represents a further decline from already low levels of trade in the past four years. Unlike what was the case some years ago, only a small portion of trade in safrole was in the form of safrole-rich oils. During the reporting period, there were only two pre-export notifications of less than 10 litres for isosafrole.

Trafficking

93. Seizures of safrole and safrole-rich oils reported through form D for 2015 were negligible. With about 75 litres of safrole seized in three incidents, Australia reported the largest safrole seizures in 2015. There were no seizures of isosafrole and no reports of suspicious or stopped shipments involving any of the three substances.

94. With regard to several seizures that were under investigation or verification at the time of the Board's last report on precursors, the Board regrets that no further

information has been forthcoming. This applies to a seizure of 2,100 litres of isosafrole reported by Namibia in 2014, for which INCB tried to determine the circumstances of the seizure and the origin of the substance. It also applies to the seizure of nearly 5,000 litres of safrole-rich oils buried in underground tanks in Cambodia, the seizure of 5 tons of unspecified amphetamine-type stimulant precursors in the Lao People's Democratic Republic near the border with Viet Nam, and the seizure of a large-scale sophisticated laboratory operation capable of producing industrial-scale volumes of MDMA in Ontario, Canada, in June 2015. **Governments are required to report seizures on form D and are requested to provide additional information on the background and circumstances of a seizure in response to INCB inquiries, with a view to supporting follow-up investigations, disseminating relevant information widely and preventing similar diversions in the future and elsewhere.**

95. Seizures of safrole and safrole-rich oils continued to be communicated through PICS in 2016. Two seizures occurred in illicit laboratories in the Netherlands; however, the amounts were small. INCB is also aware of another seizure of about 110 litres in Cambodia but has not yet been able to verify the details.

3. Use of non-scheduled substances and other trends in the illicit manufacture of amphetamine-type stimulants

96. In accordance with article 12, paragraph 12 (b), Governments are required to provide information on form D about any substance not included in Table I or Table II which is identified as having been used in illicit manufacture of narcotic drugs or psychotropic substances and which is deemed by the party to be sufficiently significant to be brought to the attention of the Board. In recent years, INCB has received such information for a number of substances used in the illicit manufacture of amphetamine-type stimulants, reflecting the diversification that has occurred in the illicit manufacture of those substances over time. **INCB commends those Governments that provided information about non-scheduled substances on form D and encourages them to consider making better use of PICS for the early sharing of such information worldwide.**

97. The following subsections provide information on non-scheduled substances and other trends in the illicit manufacture of amphetamine-type stimulants, split to the extent possible into subsections for pre-precursors for amphetamine and methamphetamine, and pre-precursors for MDMA and other "ecstasy"-type substances. A number of chemicals are required in the illicit manufacture of all amphetamine-type stimulants and even other drug types; they are included in the subsections for which the most information was available.

(a) Pre-precursors for amphetamine and methamphetamine

98. On form D for 2015, a number of countries reported seizures of substances not included in Table I or Table II of the 1988 Convention but which were identified as having been used in illicit amphetamine or methamphetamine manufacture.

99. Mexico reported an increase of almost 38 per cent in the dismantling of illicit methamphetamine laboratories (an increase from 141 dismantled laboratories in 2014 to 195 in 2015). The predominant method of illicit methamphetamine manufacture in those laboratories continued to be based on P-2-P. However, in contrast to previous years when the starting materials were mostly esters and other derivatives of phenylacetic acid, the use of the nitrostyrene method, which starts from benzaldehyde and nitroethane via, or from, the intermediary product 1-phenyl-2-nitropropene, has become increasingly common in that country. In 2015, for the first time, Mexican authorities seized more than 4,000 litres of benzaldehyde and almost 5,500 litres of 1-phenyl-2-nitropropene. In August 2016, United States authorities seized a misdeclared consignment of nearly 36 tons of benzaldehyde en route from India to Mexico.

100. The fact that more than 12 tons of iron powder were seized in Mexico in 2015 provides further evidence of an increasing use of the nitrostyrene method for illicit methamphetamine manufacture in the country. The shift in P-2-P-based manufacturing methods for the illicit manufacture of methamphetamine in North America, from the use of phenylacetic acid and its derivatives to the nitrostyrene method and use of benzaldehyde as a starting material has also been confirmed by forensic drug-profiling programmes. In the first six months of 2016, 51 per cent of selected samples analysed in the United States and found to be based on P-2-P as a chemical intermediary used the nitrostyrene method, and only 21 per cent started from phenylacetic acid and its derivatives, while ephedrine-based and pseudoephedrine-based methods had disappeared.[18]

101. INCB is concerned about indications arising in 2016 that the know-how of Mexican illicit methamphetamine laboratory operators has reached countries in Africa.

---

[18] United States Drug Enforcement Administration Special Testing Laboratory, Methamphetamine Profiling Programme, 2016.

Specifically, in March 2016, the Nigerian authorities dismantled the first industrial-scale illicit methamphetamine laboratory. The chemicals found at the laboratory, which was located in an abandoned factory in an industrial area of Delta State of Nigeria, suggested a manufacturing method based on the nitrostyrene method; four Mexican nationals were among the arrestees. The chemicals, most of which are not yet scheduled in Nigeria, were purchased from legitimate sources within the country. Investigations are ongoing.

102. In addition to Mexico, seizures of benzaldehyde were reported by five other countries, of which four also reported seizures of nitroethane and/or 1-phenyl-2-nitropropene, indicative of the nitrostyrene method for illicit amphetamine or methamphetamine manufacture. Such combined seizures were reported by the authorities of Austria, Estonia, Mexico, Poland and the Russian Federation. The incident in Austria had previously been communicated through PICS with relevant operational details; the chemicals had been imported from China via Germany. In June 2016, a seizure of 600 kg of 1-phenyl-2-nitropropene was communicated through PICS; the substance was transiting Belgium, from China to Italy.

103. After several years in which there had been no seizures of international shipments of methylamine (monomethylamine),[19] in 2015 Mexico reported the seizure of nearly 25,000 litres of methylamine upon arrival at a seaport. Seizures of methylamine were also reported by an additional six countries (Estonia, France, Guatemala, Netherlands, Poland and United States); especially in Europe, seizures may also have been related to the illicit manufacture of MDMA (see para. 116, below).

104. In 2015, Mexico also seized ammonium chloride (more than 1.8 tons) with reported links to illicit methamphetamine manufacture, as well as heroin manufacture. Although no further details were provided, ammonium chloride might have been used for the illicit manufacture of methylamine.

105. The investigation of a case of diversion of significant amounts of methylamine from shipments from the United States to Mexico, detected in 2010, was concluded in October 2015. The company in the United States was charged for knowingly exporting methylamine, a regulated chemical in the United States, without verifying the legitimacy of the transaction and for failing to report the missing shipments.

106. When methamphetamine or amphetamine is manufactured using methods starting from, or via, P-2-P, tartaric acid is needed to make the more potent form of methamphetamine. Mexico has regularly reported significant seizures of tartaric acid since 2009. In 2015, seizures amounted to nearly 5 tons; over the years, the amounts seized have ranged between 2 and 8 tons, with the exception of 2011, when nearly 60 tons were seized (see figure VI). All reports of seizures have been linked with illicit methamphetamine manufacture.

Figure VI. Seizures of chemicals associated with illicit methamphetamine manufacture reported on form D by Mexico, 2009-2015

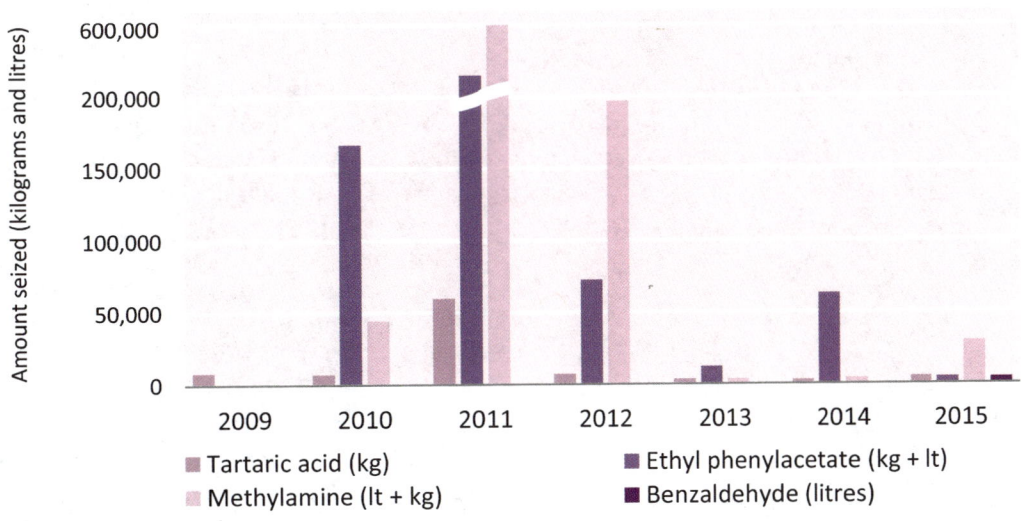

107. "Designer" precursors of amphetamine and methamphetamine were reported to have been seized in four countries. Belgium reported seizures of small amounts of unspecified P-2-P methyl glycidic acid derivatives. Authorities in the Netherlands, within a two-week period in

---

[19] Methylamine is not only a key chemical for the illicit manufacture of methamphetamine. It is also required to produce MDMA and several new psychoactive substances. Seizures in Mexico are assumed to be related to the illicit manufacture of methamphetamine.

November 2015, seized almost 3.3 tons of the sodium salt of P-2-P methyl glycidic acid (a precursor of P-2-P) when it arrived in Rotterdam. Both consignments had been declared as wallpaper glue. In one case, the consignment was mixed with more than 700 kg of the sodium salt of 3,4-MDP-2-P methyl glycidic acid (a precursor of 3,4-MDP-2-P and of "ecstasy"; see paras. 111-117, below), originating in China, transiting Hong Kong, China, and destined for the Netherlands. Additional seizures occurred in France and the Netherlands in 2016, the most significant involving almost 2.3 tons of the substance seized from a warehouse in the Netherlands in August 2016.

108. Germany reported on form D for 2015 the seizure of a mixture consisting of about 200 kg of APAA and 35 kg of APAAN. German authorities had already communicated that seizure through PICS in June 2015. APAA is not under international control and appears to have filled the gap left when APAAN, its immediate precursor, was placed in Table I of the 1988 Convention in October 2014.[20] In the first 10 months of 2016, seven additional incidents involving APAA, in amounts totalling more than 5.6 tons, were communicated through PICS, and INCB is aware of further incidents amounting to an additional 800 kg; all incidents occurred in Europe. **Governments are reminded once again of the possibility of traffickers approaching legitimate industry for customized synthesis of non-scheduled intermediaries and of the need to alert industry to that possibility.**

109. The Philippine authorities confirmed on their form D for 2015 the seizure of more than 650 kg of 1,2-dimethyl-3-phenylaziridine, an unusual chemical not under international control which is known as an intermediary product in the illicit manufacture of methamphetamine from ephedrines. However, as the Board noted in its 2015 report on precursors, the substance is also an artefact from the laboratory analysis of "chloro(pseudo)ephedrine",[21] another "designer" precursor of methamphetamine. Attempts by INCB to verify the nature of the chemical with the Philippine authorities have so far been unsuccessful.

110. Various countries in Europe, East and South-East Asia, Oceania and South America also reported other chemicals not under international control that were seized in relation to clandestine manufacture of amphetamine or methamphetamine in 2015. The substances most frequently reported included iodine and red phosphorous. Japan reported having dismantled a small-scale illicit methamphetamine manufacturing operation involving ephedrine, red phosphorous and hydrogen iodide. Instances of illicit methamphetamine manufacture using methods involving these chemicals were also reported by the authorities of Germany and New Zealand. In most of the above reports, information about the origin of the chemicals was not provided or not available.

(b) Pre-precursors for 3,4-methylenedioxymethamphetamine and related "ecstasy"-type drugs

111. In the period 2015-2016, six countries reported incidents involving pre-precursors for MDMA and related "ecstasy"-type drugs, which are not listed in Table I or Table II of the 1988 Convention. All seizures occurred in Europe and typically involved substances that could be classified as "designer" precursors, i.e., substances that are not available off-the-shelf but made specifically on demand. Overall, amounts were significantly less than just a few years ago; operational details of those seizures were typically shared through PICS.

112. Seizures of non-scheduled "ecstasy"-type precursors in amounts larger than 1 ton involved salts and esters of 3,4-MDP-2-P methyl glycidic acid (Bulgaria, Netherlands and Romania), and 3,4-(methylenedioxy)phenylacetonitrile (Netherlands). Smaller amounts of those substances were also seized in Germany and France.

113. Seizures of about 80 kg of 1-(3,4-methylenedioxyphenyl)-2-nitropropene in the Netherlands and France illustrate that illicit operators are exploring manufacturing methods for MDMA similar to those for amphetamine and methamphetamine: the substance can be considered the MDMA-precursor equivalent of 1-phenyl-2-nitropropene, indicative of the nitrostyrene method (see above).

114. Where such information was available, the substances mentioned above were typically reported to have originated in China; Hong Kong, China; or Taiwan Province of China, and to be destined for the Netherlands. Poland and Ukraine were also mentioned as destination countries. None of the substances are under international control but all are included in the INCB limited international special surveillance list. That list includes key substitute chemicals and relevant extended definitions capturing a range of derivatives and chemically related substances and is available to competent national authorities as part of the information package on the control of precursors, on the secure website of INCB.

---

[20] The first known seizure of APAA occurred in the Netherlands in December 2012 and was communicated through PICS.

[21] The term "chloro(pseudo)ephedrine" is used to reflect the fact that the substance is typically a mixture of the diastereomeric forms of what are commonly known as chloroephedrine and chloropseudoephedrine.

115. Other non-scheduled chemicals that were reported seized in 2015 included hydrogen gas and methylamine. Germany reported several thefts involving a total of 16,750 litres of compressed hydrogen gas in 335 gas cylinders from company premises in the western part of Germany, near the border with the Netherlands. Some of the stolen cylinders and a truck misused for their transport were later found in the Netherlands. Thefts of hydrogen gas continued in 2016 and operational details and the modi operandi were communicated through PICS. Hydrogen gas, which is used as a reducing agent in the illicit manufacture of a number of synthetic drugs, has also been found in numerous clandestine amphetamine and "ecstasy" laboratories in the Netherlands and elsewhere.

116. Similarly, methylamine is a chemical that is usually associated with illicit methamphetamine manufacture but that is also critical in the illicit manufacture of MDMA. For example, the Netherlands reported seizures in 2015 of methylamine totalling slightly more than 10,000 litres. All seizures were made in illicit laboratories, typically manufacturing MDMA and occasionally synthetic cathinones, or in associated warehouses. Seizures of methylamine also continued in 2016, typically in illicit laboratories in the Netherlands.

117. INCB commends the Governments that share information about non-scheduled pre-precursors, especially those Governments that share such information early, through PICS, to enable the authorities of other countries involved as source, transit or destination countries to initiate the requisite investigations. This applies in particular to the Netherlands (accounting for more than 30 per cent of all incidents in 2015 and 2016) and other European countries, which thus provided a starting point for follow-up and operational cooperation, and helped to raise awareness of new developments.

B. Substances used in the illicit manufacture of cocaine

118. With Colombia accounting for more than 60 per cent of global coca bush cultivation, changes in that country have significant implications for the global supply of cocaine hydrochloride. Following an increase of 44 per cent in 2014, the area under coca bush cultivation in that country increased by another 39 per cent in 2015. Potential production of cocaine hydrochloride is estimated to have increased even more in 2015, by nearly 46 per cent, compared with the previous year. In Bolivia (Plurinational State of) and Peru, the area under coca bush cultivation is reported to have slightly decreased, by 1 per cent and 6.1 per cent, respectively; the corresponding figures of potential production of sun-dried coca leaves have decreased by 2 per cent in Bolivia (Plurinational State of) and 4.5 per cent in Peru.

1. Potassium permanganate

119. Potassium permanganate is a key chemical used in the illicit manufacture of cocaine. It is traded and used widely as a disinfecting agent and for water purification and is an important reagent in synthetic organic chemistry. A minimum of about 145 tons of the substance are required annually for illicit cocaine manufacture in coca-producing countries.[22] While coca-producing countries only account for a limited proportion of legitimate international trade in potassium permanganate, a significant proportion of global seizures of potassium permanganate is reported by those countries. There are also significant seizures reported outside coca-producing regions; however, no specific reference to illicit cocaine manufacture was made in connection with those seizures. In the continued absence of any notable diversions of potassium permanganate from legitimate international trade reported to the Board, illicit manufacture of the substance and diversion from domestic distribution channels with subsequent smuggling, including across international borders, remain the major sources of potassium permanganate for illicit purposes.

Licit trade

120. Between 1 November 2015 and 1 November 2016, there were nearly 1,520 pre-export notifications for potassium permanganate, totalling nearly 25,000 tons, sent by the authorities of 29 exporting countries to the authorities in 128 importing countries. As in previous years, the three coca-producing countries in South America — Bolivia (Plurinational State of), Colombia and Peru — only accounted for about 1.5 per cent (slightly more than 240 tons) of the amount of potassium permanganate notified through the PEN Online system. Other countries in South America accounted for imports amounting to another 950 tons of the substance; none of those countries exported or re-exported any potassium permanganate.

---

[22] Based on the averages of low-end estimates for the period 2011-2014 by UNODC of the potential manufacture of 100 per cent pure cocaine, as published in *World Drug Report 2016* (see annex, p. vi), and using the approximate low-end potassium permanganate quantities contained in annex IV to the present report. Note that potential cocaine hydrochloride manufacture in Colombia increased by 46 per cent in 2015 compared with 2014 (UNODC and Government of Colombia, *Colombia: Monitoreo de Territorios Afectados por Cultivos Ilícitos 2015* (Bogota, July 2016), p. 11.

121. Pakistan reported stopped shipments of potassium permanganate on form D — a total of four stopped shipments, amounting to about 66 tons; those imports were reported to have been stopped for administrative reasons. Other countries reporting stopped shipments of potassium permanganate were Canada and Spain; however, the amounts were significantly smaller.

Trafficking

122. Fifteen countries reported seizures of potassium permanganate, totalling nearly 140 tons, on form D for 2015. Of the three coca-producing countries, Colombia accounted for the largest amount (nearly 58 tons) reported. However, levels of seizures in Colombia in 2015 were only about one third of the amount seized in 2014.[23] Significant seizures of potassium permanganate were also reported by Uzbekistan (32.7 tons), China (31.6 tons) and Kazakhstan (13.4 tons); information on the circumstances and reasons for those seizures was usually not provided. Seizures of more than 1 ton were reported by Slovakia and Venezuela (Bolivarian Republic of). The authorities of the Bolivarian Republic of Venezuela informed that almost the entire amount was seized in three illicit laboratories, thus providing further evidence for cocaine manufacture outside the three coca-producing countries. Within Colombia, the majority of the 236 cocaine crystallization laboratories (conducting the final conversion into cocaine hydrochloride) dismantled in 2015 were located in three departments: Norte de Santander (58), near the border with the Bolivarian Republic of Venezuela, and Cauca (41) and Nariño (38) in the south. **INCB reiterates its warning about the possibility of illicit cocaine manufacture and processing/reprocessing, and the related precursor trafficking, in countries outside the traditional coca-producing regions and along trafficking routes, and the need to address such developments collectively at the regional and international levels.**

123. In 2015, as a result of the significant amounts of potassium permanganate seized outside South America, the proportion of global seizures of that chemical that was seized in that region dropped to 43 per cent; within South America, the total amount of potassium permanganate seized in Bolivia (Plurinational State of) and Colombia together, 862 kg, accounted for 99 per cent of all seizures in that region (see figure VII).

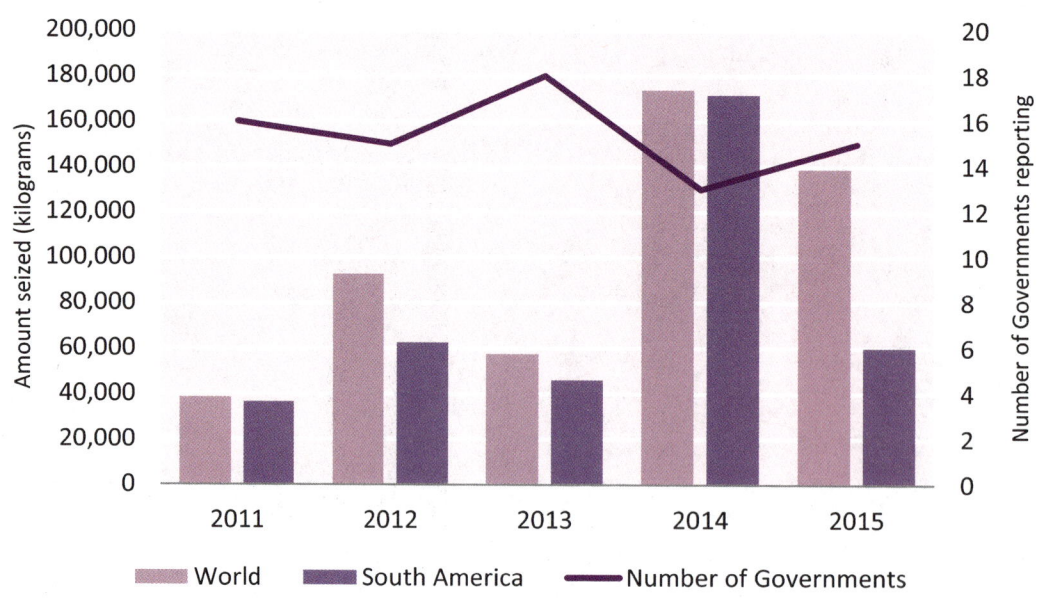

Figure VII. Seizures of potassium permanganate reported by Governments on form D, 2011-2015

124. Seizures of potassium permanganate in South American countries and Uzbekistan were reported to have mostly originated from domestic sources, while seizures in countries in other regions, for which information was available, originated in foreign countries. Colombian authorities also continued to encounter the illicit manufacture of potassium

---

[23] As in the past, the Government of Colombia indicated that the reported amounts did not include seizures of potassium permanganate in the form of solutions, as concentrations are usually not known.

permanganate from internationally non-scheduled chemicals (see paras. 126-131, below). There were 12 such facilities dismantled in 2015, up from 9 in 2014 and 3 in 2013.

125. Additional seizures of potassium permanganate were also communicated through PICS in 2016.

2. Use of non-scheduled substances and other trends in the illicit manufacture of cocaine

126. As in previous years, several countries in South America and elsewhere reported seizures of a variety of chemicals not under international control used in the processing, further refinement (after trafficking) or adulteration of cocaine. Those chemicals included (a) alternative solvents for the extraction of cocaine base from coca leaves and for the conversion of cocaine base into cocaine hydrochloride, (b) chemicals used in the illicit manufacture of internationally controlled precursors, and (c) chemicals used for improving the efficiency of cocaine processing, for example, by reducing the volume of chemicals needed and/or the processing time. Several of these alternative chemicals that are not under international control are, however, under national control in the countries concerned; they are known to have been used in illicit drug manufacture for many years and have partly replaced some chemicals under international control, in particular substances in Table II of the 1988 Convention. Furthermore, improved processing techniques, and recycling and reuse have resulted in reduced requirements for Table II acids and solvents. Where such information was provided, in the majority of cases, these chemicals were reported to have originated from domestic sources.

127. Significant amounts of such chemicals were reported on form D by the authorities of the three coca-producing countries, Bolivia (Plurinational State of), Colombia and Peru, as well as other countries in South America. Colombia reported seizures of 23 of the 25 substances under national control. The Plurinational State of Bolivia reported 28 internationally non-scheduled chemicals and Peru reported 22 substances. However, with the exception of the Bolivarian Republic of Venezuela, the amounts seized were generally much smaller than in 2014. For example, seizures of potassium manganate, a precursor of potassium permanganate, in Colombia amounted to just 785 kg in 2015, down from 4.5 tons in 2014; those seizures were reported to have been made at four illicit potassium permanganate-manufacturing locations. No seizures of manganese dioxide, another precursor of potassium permanganate, were reported in 2015 (see figure VIII).

Figure VIII. Seizures of potassium permanganate and its precursors, as reported on form D by Colombia, 2006-2015

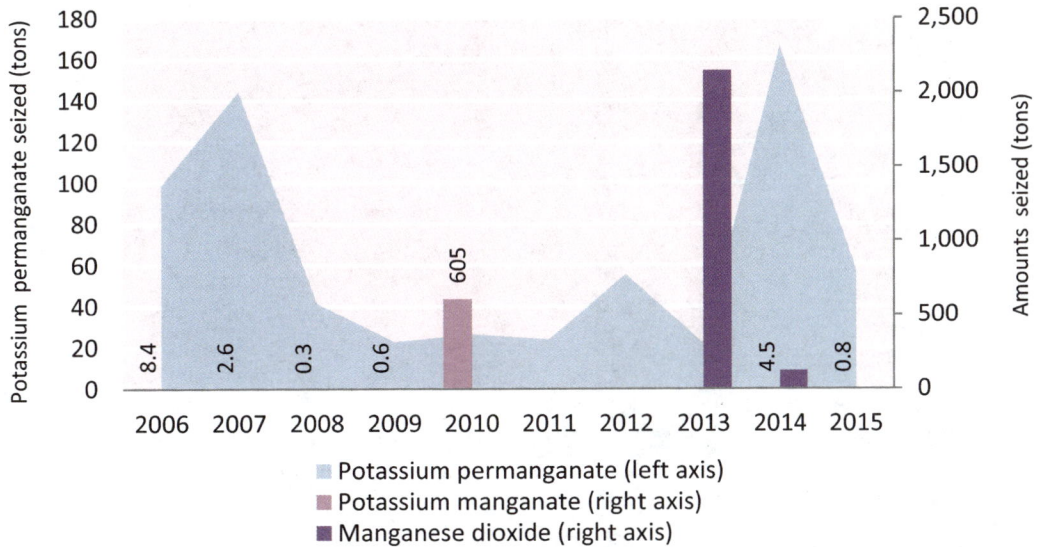

128. Significant seizures of sodium hypochlorite, a substance that can be used as a substitute for potassium permanaganate in the purification of coca paste, have regularly been reported on form D by the authorities of Bolivia (Plurinational State of) and Peru. In 2015, such seizures amounted to more than 20 tons in the Plurinational State of Bolivia and nearly 10 tons in Peru. Seizures of the substance have never been reported by Colombia.

129. Seizures of urea, a chemical that is used in the extraction step to generate ammonia,[24] also dropped significantly, mainly because Colombia, which had reported seizures of more than 3,000 tons in 2013 and 2014, did not report any seizures in 2015. Similarly, seizures in the Plurinational State of Bolivia

___

[24] Urea is also used as fertilizer in coca bush cultivation, and could also be used to produce explosives.

in 2015 were down to 240 kg, falling from more than 3 tons a year earlier. By contrast, seizures in 11 incidents in the Bolivarian Republic of Venezuela, totalling nearly 142 tons in 2015, were almost five times the amount of 2014, but still less than in 2011 and 2012.

130. Sodium metabisulfite is a reducing agent that is used to standardize the oxidation level of cocaine base obtained from different sources prior to further processing. It is not under international control but is included in the INCB limited international special surveillance list. Seizures of sodium metabisulfite, which have almost exclusively been reported by countries in South America, show a steady increase, especially in the past three years (see figure IX). In 2015, seizures were reported, in descending order, by the authorities of Colombia (103.3 tons, up from 54 tons in 2014), the Plurinational State of Bolivia (16.7 tons, about the same level as in 2014) and the Bolivarian Republic of Venezuela (3.6 tons, up from 1.9 tons). Seizures of sodium metabisulfite also continued in 2016, with incidents in illicit laboratories in Bolivia (Plurinational State of) and Colombia communicated via PICS.

Figure IX. Seizures of sodium metabisulfite, as reported on form D, 2008-2015

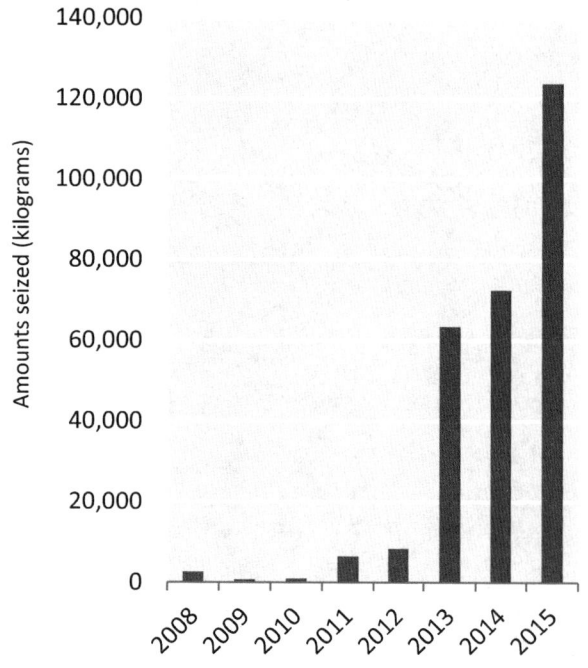

131. Calcium chloride is another chemical used to increase the efficiency of cocaine processing. Specifically, as a drying agent for solvents, it is used as part of the conversion of cocaine into cocaine hydrochloride. It is also used as part of the recycling and reuse of solvents. In 2015, seizures of calcium chloride in amounts larger than 1 ton were reported on form D by the authorities of Bolivia (Plurinational State of) (18.6 tons, up from 13 tons in 2014) and Colombia (81.9 tons, up from 28.3 tons in 2014). Several other countries reported seizures of the substance although, with the exception of the Bolivarian Republic of Venezuela (575 kg) and Spain (500 kg), in amounts not exceeding 100 kg. As for most other non-scheduled chemicals, information on the origin of calcium chloride was usually not provided.

C. Substances used in the illicit manufacture of heroin

1. Acetic anhydride

132. Acetic anhydride is one of the most widely traded substances in Table I of the 1988 Convention and it is the key chemical in the illicit manufacture of heroin. However, acetic anhydride is also required in the illicit manufacture of amphetamine and methamphetamine, namely in instances where the manufacturing process starts from phenylacetic acid or phenylacetic acid derivatives (see annex IV). While, therefore, seizures of acetic anhydride in Afghanistan and neighbouring countries, as well as in other heroin-producing regions, are typically associated with illicit heroin manufacture, seizures of the substance in Mexico and neighbouring countries might be attributed to the illicit manufacture of either heroin, or methamphetamine from phenylacetic acid derivatives.

Licit trade

133. Between 1 November 2015 and 1 November 2016, there were almost 1,580 pre-export notifications for shipments of acetic anhydride sent by the authorities of 24 exporting countries and territories to 85 importing countries and territories; those shipments involved a total of 482 million litres of acetic anhydride.[25]

134. Traffickers' attempts to divert acetic anhydride from international trade have been rather rare in past years. In 2016, a shipment of 18,500 litres of acetic anhydride to the Islamic Republic of Iran, about which the Italian authorities sent a notification through PEN Online, was suspended at the request of the Iranian regulatory authorities because the proposed importer in the Islamic Republic of Iran was not authorized to import the substance.

---

[25] This does not include trade among the individual States members of the European Union.

135. Neither the importing nor the exporting country informed INCB whether the shipment was not allowed to proceed because of administrative reasons or whether it was an actual attempt by traffickers to divert acetic anhydride. Thorough investigation into suspicious transactions and other irregularities in legitimate trade, such as in the above-mentioned case, is very important. Suspending the delivery of a suspicious precursor shipment alone, without further law enforcement investigation, is not enough, as experience has shown that the persons behind the suspicious order may continue looking for acetic anhydride in other source countries.

Trafficking

136. Since 2010, the total global seizures of acetic anhydride, reported on form D, amounted to more than 695,000 litres. China, Afghanistan and Mexico, in that order, were the countries reporting the largest volumes of the substance (see figure X).

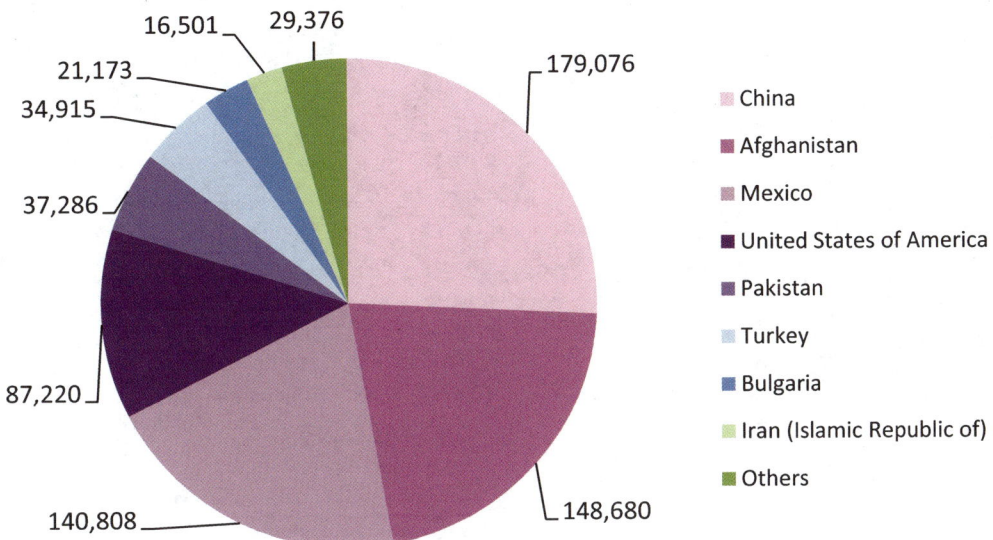

Figure X. Seizures of acetic anhydride (in litres), as reported on form D, 2010-2015

137. Seventeen countries and territories reported seizures of acetic anhydride on form D for 2015. The largest volume was reported by China (more than 11,000 litres), followed by Pakistan (about 5,300 litres) and Turkey (more than 4,400 litres). Seizures of more than 1,000 litres were also reported by Afghanistan, Argentina, Austria and Mexico. Myanmar reported having seized 60 litres of acetic anhydride in 2015, the first such report by that country in more than five years. **The lack of reported seizures of acetic anhydride and other chemicals required to manufacture heroin remains a concern worldwide.**

138. With regard to Afghanistan and countries in Central Asia that share a border with Afghanistan, the situation regarding acetic anhydride trafficking has not changed from the last reporting period. The Board noted the continued lack of seizures of acetic anhydride reported by Tajikistan, Turkmenistan and Uzbekistan on form D, a situation that has prevailed for the past 15 years.

139. In Afghanistan, the sharp decline in seizures of acetic anhydride continued throughout 2015 as well as the first half of 2016. The total volume of acetic anhydride seized in Afghanistan in 2015 was 3,760 litres, or just about half the volume reported in 2014, and thus continuing the declining trend, at a year-on-year rate of 50 per cent, that had started in 2011 (see figure XI). According to data provided by Afghanistan on form D for 2015, the acetic anhydride seized in that country was trafficked through the country's border with the Islamic Republic of Iran, in 18 incidents.

140. Although the Iranian authorities did not provide any seizure data on form D for 2015, INCB understands from information published on the Iranian customs authorities website that in 2015, the country's customs authorities seized two large consignments, of 9.3 tons and 17.6 tons of acetic anhydride, destined for Afghanistan. Through PICS, INCB is also aware of a further consignment seized by Iranian customs authorities in February 2016 involving 11.5 tons of acetic anhydride; the consignment purportedly originated in Taiwan Province of China and was also destined for Afghanistan. In 2016, there were additional media reports about seizures of further amounts of acetic anhydride or other chemicals in the Islamic Republic of Iran; these seizures could not be confirmed with the Iranian authorities by the time of finalizing the present report.

Figure XI. Seizures of acetic anhydride, as reported on form D by Afghanistan, 2010-2015

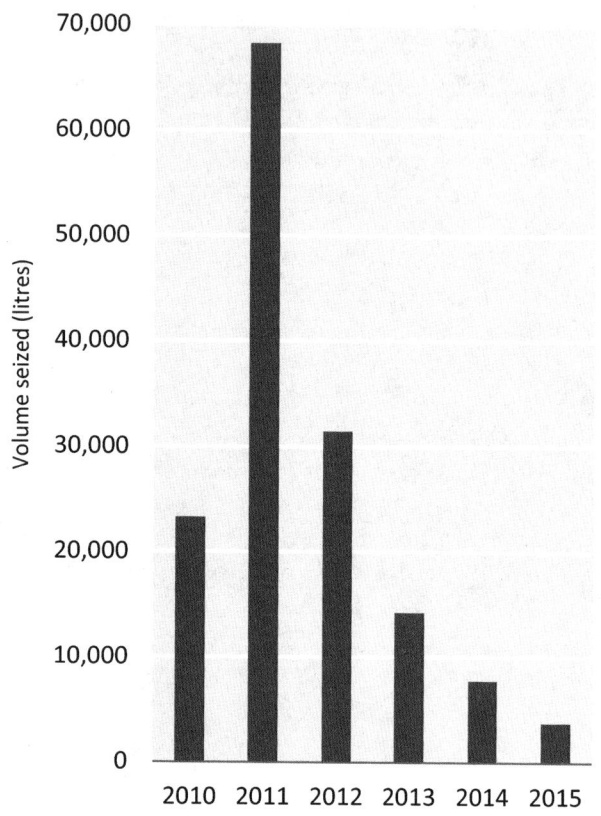

141. Also in early 2016, the authorities of Pakistan communicated through PICS a seizure of more than 20,000 litres (21.7 tons) of acetic anhydride. The seized substance was declared at customs as a shipment of glacial acetic acid from the United Republic of Tanzania. For several reasons, the seizure is one of the most salient incidents involving acetic anhydride in the past few years. Of particular importance is the almost real-time communication of the seizure by the customs authorities of Pakistan through PICS, which enabled the quick launch of backtracking investigations in several countries. These investigations resulted in the identification of a suspected country of origin of the seized substance (China), a point of diversion (United Republic of Tanzania) and the modus operandi used by the traffickers. **The swift and pragmatic cooperation with and between the relevant authorities of China and the United Republic of Tanzania resulted in the prevention of the diversion of further amounts of acetic anhydride to companies in the United Republic of Tanzania.**

142. The investigations assisted in the identification of weaknesses in the control system in the United Republic of Tanzania. They also confirmed the Board's suspicion and previous alerts regarding the potential use of glacial acetic acid to mislabel, misdeclare or otherwise disguise shipments of contraband acetic anhydride.

143. In addition to the above seizure, the Pakistani authorities communicated through PICS three additional seizures of acetic anhydride amounting to nearly 18,000 litres in the first 10 months of 2016, including a seizure of about 15,000 litres of acetic anhydride smuggled from Hong Kong, China, and misdeclared as formic acid. Overall, the Board is pleased to note that reported seizures of acetic anhydride in both the Islamic Republic of Iran and Pakistan have finally started to increase from the relatively low levels observed in previous years.

144. In India, another country in the vicinity of heroin manufacture sites in West Asia, the total volume of seized acetic anhydride has amounted to less than 800 litres since 2010. INCB is aware of a seizure of nearly 2,500 litres of acetic anhydride in India in April 2016. However, as the seizure was made in connection with a major case of diversion of ephedrines (see para. 69, above), it is possible that the substance may have been intended for purposes other than diversion into illicit heroin manufacture.

145. INCB has also previously noted a lack of information about the sources of acetic anhydride feeding illicit heroin manufacture in other parts of the world. For example, according to the UNODC *World Drug Report 2016*, the potential production of oven-dry opium in Myanmar averaged around 700 tons annually in the period 2011-2015, with a peak of 870 tons in 2013; it has averaged about 260 tons per year in Mexico in the period 2011-2014, with a recent upward trend. The corresponding figures for potential manufacture of heroin are 70 tons (Myanmar) and 26 tons (Mexico),[26] amounts which would require about 122,000 litres (Myanmar) and 45,000 litres (Mexico) of acetic anhydride.

2. Use of non-scheduled substances and other trends in the illicit manufacture of heroin

146. The non-scheduled chemicals most frequently associated with illicit heroin manufacture are ammonium chloride, commonly used as part of the extraction of morphine from opium, and glacial acetic acid, which has long been suspected of being used as a possible cover load to conceal contraband acetic anhydride, as well as in the acetylation of morphine to yield heroin, likely mixed with acetic anhydride. Neither chemical is under international control but both are in the limited international special

---

[26] Assuming that all opium produced is converted into heroin using a conversion ratio of opium to heroin (of unknown purity) of 10:1.

surveillance list and, according to information available to INCB, are under national control in a number of countries and territories (21 countries and territories in the case of glacial acetic acid and 8 countries and territories in the case of ammonium chloride). Another acetylating agent, acetyl chloride, is controlled in 17 countries and territories.

147. For several years, the largest seizures of ammonium chloride have been reported on form D by Afghanistan (see figure XII). In 2015, four countries reported seizures of ammonium chloride. The largest seizures were reported by Mexico (1.8 tons), with links to illicit heroin but also methamphetamine laboratories (see para. 104, above). Seizures in Afghanistan amounted to slightly more than 1.2 tons, a decrease of almost 95 per cent compared with the amounts reported in 2014; seizures in other countries did not exceed 25 kg. A seizure of nearly 1.3 tons of ammonium chloride at the Pakistan/Afghanistan border in March 2016 was communicated through PICS by the authorities of Pakistan. Notable seizures of glacial acetic acid were reported only by Mexico, the Netherlands and countries in South America, but without any reference to illicit heroin manufacture.

Figure XII. Seizures of ammonium chloride reported on form D by Afghanistan and other countries, 2011-2015

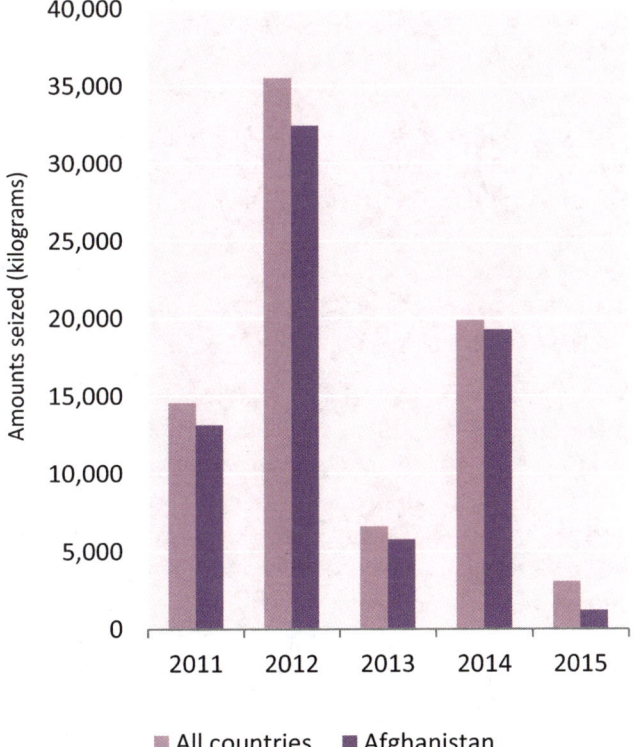

D. Substances used in the illicit manufacture of other narcotic drugs and psychotropic substances

1. Ergot alkaloids and lysergic acid

Licit trade

148. There is comparatively limited international trade in ergot alkaloids (ergometrine and ergotamine and their salts), which are used in the treatment of migraines and as an oxytocic in obstetrics. Between 1 November 2015 and 1 November 2016, 341 shipments of ergot alkaloids, totalling 1,530 kg, were notified by 15 exporting countries to 44 importing countries; the volumes involved and the number of pre-export notifications are similar to last year. In addition, there were three pre-export notifications for lysergic acid, totalling 0.2 grams.

Trafficking

149. Reports on form D of seizures of precursors of lysergic acid diethylamide (LSD) continue to be infrequent and in small amounts, even considering the potency of the LSD end-product. In 2015, Australia reported having seized 281 grams of ergotamine in six incidents; Canada reported the seizure of about 30 grams of ergotamine and small amounts of lysergic acid; and India seized 470 grams of lysergic acid as well as additional amounts in liquid form, in 26 instances. Information about the origin of the seized substances was not provided.

2. *N*-Acetylanthranilic acid and anthranilic acid

Licit trade

150. *N*-Acetylanthranilic acid and anthranilic acid are precursors that can be used for the illicit manufacture of methaqualone, a sedative-hypnotic which is also known, in reference to its former brand names, as "quaalude" and "mandrax". While anthranilic acid is traded widely in industrial quantities, trade in *N*-acetylanthranilic acid is limited to small amounts, typically for analytical and research purposes. Between 1 November 2015 and 1 November 2016, there were nearly 320 pre-export notifications sent by 9 exporting countries to 40 importing countries for shipments of anthranilic acid. Those shipments together amounted to more than 1,450 tons; major exporters were China and India, and the major importers were Germany and the United Kingdom of Great Britain and Northern Ireland. By contrast, the five pre-export notifications for shipments of *N*-acetylanthranilic acid did not exceed 150 grams.

Trafficking

151. For the third consecutive year, China was the only country to report significant seizures of anthranilic acid on form D, amounting to more than 9.5 tons in 2015. Total global seizures of N-acetylanthranilic acid since 2010 have amounted to just 15 kg. In 2015, China was the only country reporting seizures of that substance, in a negligible amount. The origin and circumstances of the seizures were not provided.

152. Although the official website of the South African Police Service regularly reports seizures of suspected methaqualone tablets, locally known as "mandrax", as well as alleged laboratories illicitly manufacturing such tablets, very little corresponding precursor seizure information was provided through form D. In 2015, the South African authorities reported a seizure of 37,000 litres of *ortho*-toluidine, a methaqualone precursor not under international control but included in the limited international special surveillance list. **INCB wishes to encourage all Governments to make every effort to provide details of, and confirm, relevant seizures when so requested by the Board. It is only through the sharing of such information that weaknesses in control systems can be identified in a timely manner and be successfully addressed.**

E. Solvents and acids used in the illicit manufacture of various narcotic drugs and psychotropic substances

1. Solvents and acids in Table II of the 1988 Convention

153. Acids, bases and solvents are required throughout various stages of nearly all illicit drug manufacture. There are two acids, hydrochloric acid and sulphuric acid, as well as four solvents, acetone, ethyl ether, methyl ethyl ketone and toluene, included in Table II of the 1988 Convention. A number of acids and solvents, as well as key bases, are included in the INCB limited international special surveillance list; country-specific and region-specific chemicals are under national control in various countries.

154. A total of 36 countries and territories reported on form D seizures of Table II acids and solvents in 2015, while 14 countries reported seizures of non-scheduled alternate chemicals. The majority of the countries reporting non-scheduled alternate chemicals were in South America; countries in Europe included the Netherlands, Poland and Spain, and, in South-East Asia, Malaysia and Thailand.

155. Given that illicit heroin and cocaine processing operations are, on average, much larger than illicit synthetic drug manufacturing operations, the largest amounts of those chemicals traditionally used to be seized in countries in which plant-based drug manufacture is known to occur. However, as illicit synthetic drug operations increase in size and reporting of the chemicals seized in illicit laboratories in some regions improves, the range of countries reporting Table II chemicals is also increasing.[27]

156. Acetone was the solvent that was seized in the largest volume in 2015; of the total volume, Colombia reported having seized more than 60 per cent (nearly 615,000 litres), followed by the Bolivarian Republic of Venezuela (more than 200,000 litres). The Netherlands ranked fifth, with nearly 21,000 litres. Seizures of acetone of more than 5,000 litres were also reported by Argentina, Bolivia (Plurinational State of), China, Mexico, Peru and Uzbekistan. Colombia also ranked second and third of all countries reporting seizures of, respectively, ethyl ether (11,700 litres) and toluene (56,000 litres); the largest seizures of ethyl ether and toluene were reported in 2015 by, respectively, the Plurinational State of Bolivia (12,300 litres) and China (nearly 92,000 litres). Seizures of toluene above 20,000 litres were also reported by Argentina, Mexico and Ukraine.

157. Seizures of methyl ethyl ketone, a chemical included in Table II of the 1988 Convention primarily because of its use in illicit cocaine processing, were insignificant in coca-producing countries; Spain (1,061 litres) followed by China (726 litres) and the Netherlands (409 litres), reported the largest seizures of methyl ethyl ketone. While seizures in Spain were likely linked to illicit cocaine processing, seizures in China (726 litres) and the Netherlands (409 litres), were more likely connected with synthetic drug manufacture. In cocaine processing in countries in South America, a range of substitute solvents are known to have largely replaced the use of methyl ethyl ketone (see para. 163, below).

158. Thirty-two countries reported seizures of hydrochloric and/or sulphuric acid in 2015. The largest volumes of hydrochloric acid were reported by China (more than 565,000 litres), Brazil (nearly 375,000 litres), Colombia (more than 211,000 litres) and Mexico (more than 188,000 litres); Argentina, Belarus, the Netherlands and Venezuela (Bolivarian Republic of) reported seizures of more than 15,000 litres. With regard to sulphuric acid, Brazil, Colombia and China, in that order, reported the largest volumes, each larger than 150,000 litres; seizures in

---

[27] See annex IV for the approximate quantities of Table II acids and solvents required for the illicit manufacture of cocaine or heroin.

Afghanistan, Bolivia (Plurinational State of), the Netherlands and Peru ranged between 15,000 litres and 52,000 litres.

159. Not unexpectedly, seizures of acids and solvents in Table II of the 1988 Convention were also reported in connection with illicit synthetic drug manufacture. For example, the authorities of Czechia reported seizures of hydrochloric acid, sulphuric acid and toluene in the small-scale illicit methamphetamine laboratories detected in that country. All chemicals were sourced domestically, typically from specialized drug stores from which those chemicals are easily available, as most are widely used for different household purposes.

160. Another continuing trend, in the United States, is methamphetamine entering the country in liquid form. The recrystallization or recovery process is not complicated but requires a significant amount of solvents such as acetone.

2. Solvents not included in Table II of the 1988 Convention

161. Solvents not included in Table II of the 1988 Convention have regularly been reported on form D, most frequently and in the largest diversity, by countries in South America, where they are often under national control.

162. Of those countries, Colombia has the most consistent record of such seizures. In 2015, Colombia reported having seized a range of acetate solvents, including butyl acetate (15,255 litres), ethyl acetate (106,614 litres), isobutyl acetate (127,334 litres), isopropyl acetate (30,745 litres), *n*-propyl acetate (20,305 litres) (see figure XIII). These solvents all substitute for Table II solvents, especially in the final crystallization step, when cocaine base is converted into cocaine hydrochloride. Another solvent that can be used in that step that was reported seized in Colombia is methyl isobutyl ketone (9,476 litres). Where information was available, the substitute solvents were obtained from domestic sources; they are all under control in Colombia.

Figure XIII. Seizures of solvents in Table II[a] and non-scheduled acetate solvents, as reported on form D by Colombia, 2006-2015

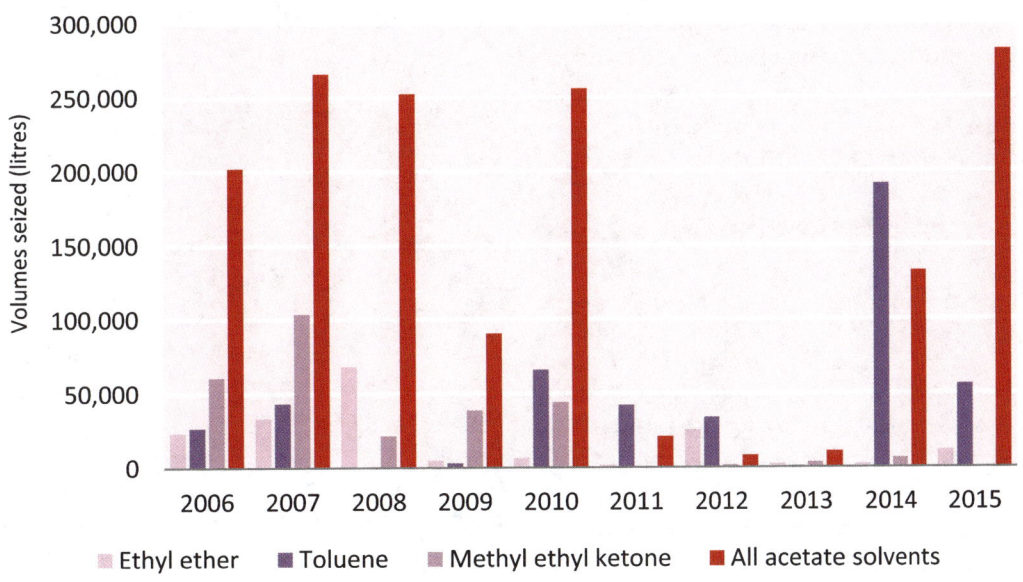

[a] Excluding acetone.

163. Countries in South America also regularly report a range of other solvents or solvent mixtures that are predominantly employed in the extraction of cocaine from coca leaves. They include various hydrocarbon solvent mixtures, such as common thinners, kerosene, diesel and various types of gasoline. Several countries reported seizures of a variety of non-scheduled chemicals used in the processing/reprocessing, refinement and/or cutting of cocaine. Such incidents, often illicit laboratory incidents outside the three coca-growing countries, were reported, for example, by Chile and Spain.

164. Using forensic analysis to determine the solvents used in illicit cocaine processing, namely those used in the final crystallization step, can help to identify linkages between samples of seized cocaine hydrochloride, establish processing trends and, hence, provide valuable information for regulatory controls.

165. Seizures of significant volumes of non-scheduled solvents outside South America appear to be more often individual incidents rather than part of a trend. For example, Thailand reported on form D for 2015 having seized 20,000 litres of methylene chloride (dichloromethane) in connection with suspected illicit methamphetamine manufacture in Myanmar.

166. Acids and solvents included in Table II of the 1988 Convention, as well as alternate chemicals not under international control also continued to be communicated through PICS in 2016.

F. Substances not in Table I or Table II of the 1988 Convention that are used in the illicit manufacture of other narcotic drugs and psychotropic substances or substances of abuse not under international control

167. Although at lower levels, in 2015, Governments also continued to use form D to report seizures of a variety of substances not in Table I or Table II of the 1988 Convention that can be used in the manufacture of other narcotic drugs and psychotropic substances, precursors, or substances of abuse not under international control, including new psychoactive substances. INCB has also been made aware of such information through PICS. However, in some instances the same information was subsequently not included in the annual submission of form D.

1. Precursors of fentanyl

168. INCB is aware, through PICS, of a number of incidents involving precursors of fentanyl, a substance in Schedule I of the 1961 Convention, in Canada and the United States. Specifically, Canadian authorities seized 1.5 kg of NPP, together with a variety of other chemicals, in an illicit laboratory near Edmonton in Canada's western province of Alberta in December 2015. At around the same time, United States' authorities reported seizures of shipments of ANPP entering the United States through Los Angeles International Airport. Together with seizures made following a controlled delivery, the incidents involved a total of 78 kg of ANPP. In September 2016, authorities in the United Kingdom seized two consignments, of 500 grams each, of NPP. Investigations in all countries are ongoing.

169. The seizures of fentanyl precursors provide evidence of the illicit manufacture of fentanyl in North America as one potential source of the drug considered to be responsible for the largest increase in drug overdose deaths in the United States and Canada in recent years. In addition, authorities of both countries have also encountered the smuggling of illicitly manufactured fentanyl and other synthetic "designer" opioids into their territories. The amounts of drugs and precursors seized should be viewed in the light of the potency of synthetic opioids, as 1 kg of such synthetic opioids may provide several million street doses. It is in that context that the United States authorities have initiated the process of including the two chemicals in Table I of the 1988 Convention (see para. 8, above) and that the United States Drug Enforcement Administration is currently monitoring the shipments of fentanyl and fentanyl analogue precursors, as well as the emergence of synthetic opioids. INCB welcomes the measures to address new developments in precursor trafficking taken by Governments at the national level. However, INCB also wishes to highlight once again the importance of the early sharing of information about emerging chemicals and new trends in precursor trafficking at the global level and encourages all Governments to make better use of PICS and the form D for this purpose.

2. Precursors of *gamma*-hydroxybutyric acid

170. *gamma*-Butyrolactone (GBL) can be used in the illicit manufacture of *gamma*-hydroxybutyric acid (GHB) but is also used as a drug per se, as it is metabolized in the body into GHB, following ingestion; it is often not possible to ascertain whether seized GBL was intended for conversion to GHB or consumption as GBL. 1,4-Butanediol is a precursor of GBL and a pre-precursor of GHB. In 2015, nine European countries reported seizures of GBL. The largest seizures were reported by Latvia (1,057 litres) followed by Norway (930 litres in 68 incidents); Norway was also named as the destination of the amount of the substance seized in Germany. Seizures outside Europe were negligible. 1,4-Butanediol was only reported seized by Australia, although amounts were small. Information about the origin of the seized substances and the shipping mode was usually not provided; one country mentioned international courier services.

171. Seizures of GBL continued in 2016 and were communicated through both PICS and the Project Ion Incident Communication System (IONICS). They included three incidents in Poland, including a bulk seizure of 2.8 tons. While smaller volumes of between 100 millilitres and 5 litres were typically shipped by courier service, mislabelled as cleaning agents, to private consignees, the seizure of the bulk amount was effected at a Polish seaport. Additional seizures of GBL were communicated by PICS users in Australia, Belgium, France, the Netherlands, the United Kingdom and the United

States, involving amounts between 1 litre and 1,000 litres; the seizures of the substance were typically effected at airports or post/mail/parcel facilities — where the substance had been mislabelled or misdeclared; there were also seizures at seaports and at a warehouse.

3. Precursors of ketamine

172. In its annual report on drug control,[28] China reported 118 cases of illicit ketamine manufacture in 2015, an increase of 12.4 per cent compared with 2014. Cases of illicit manufacture also included the manufacture of two chemical intermediaries of ketamine: "hydroxylimine" and o-chlorophenyl cyclopentyl ketone.

173. In August 2016, Malaysian authorities dismantled an industrial-scale illicit ketamine laboratory estimated to have produced more than 100 kg of ketamine since October 2015, in production cycles of about a week, each with a capacity of 5 kg to 10 kg. The lengthy production cycle and chemicals found in the laboratory suggest that the illicit operators, which included Malaysian and Indian nationals, used basic chemicals and not any of the chemical intermediaries of ketamine that had been reported as starting materials in other ketamine laboratories in the recent past. Investigations suggest that the chemicals and glassware were smuggled from India.

4. Precursors of new psychoactive substances, including substances recently scheduled under the 1961 Convention or the 1971 Convention

174. Following the inclusion, effective 4 November 2015, of mephedrone in Schedule II of the 1971 Convention, INCB has become aware of an increasing number of incidents involving precursors of that substance that are not under international control. On form D for 2015, Poland reported seizures of chemicals associated with the illicit manufacture of mephedrone, and the dismantling of a medium-size laboratory. Seizures of the mephedrone precursor 2-bromo-4'-methylpropiophenone were made in clandestine laboratories in the Netherlands in November 2015. Additional incidents involving the substance were communicated by the authorities in the Netherlands and France, in amounts totalling nearly 80 kg; in those incidents, the substance originated in China, and transited France en route to Poland or Ukraine, or transited Germany destined for the Netherlands.

175. Seizures involving precursors of other new psychoactive substances also continued to be communicated through PICS in 2016, such as precursors for 2-fluoroamphetamine or 2-fluoromethamphetamine and 4-chloroamphetamine or 4-chloromethamphetamine.

5. Precursors of other drugs and cutting agents

176. Following seizures of the substance in the Netherlands in 2014, the authorities of Latvia reported having seized about 1.8 kg of 4-methoxy-P-2-P, the non-scheduled equivalent of P-2-P used in the illicit manufacture of para-methoxyamphetamine (PMA) and para-methoxymethamphetamine (PMMA) in 2015; no further information was provided.

177. Estonia reported on form D for 2015 the seizure of 43 kg of lithium aluminium hydride, in connection with the illicit manufacture of three amphetamine-type stimulants under international control (trimethoxyamphetamine (TMA), 4-bromo-2,5-dimethoxyphenethylamine (2C-B) and 2,5-dimethoxyamphetamine (DMA)).

178. The United States reported on form D for 2015 the dismantling of an illicit phencyclidine (PCP) laboratory in California and the seizure of a number of chemicals, including ethyl ether, sodium bisulfite and sodium cyanide. This and previous PCP laboratories were also communicated through PICS.

179. A number of countries also continued to report seizures of cutting agents (adulterants and diluents), often in amounts of several hundred kilograms. Such reports occur in connection with all types of drugs. The substance most frequently encountered as a cutting agent in connection with different types of drugs is caffeine, reported in 2015 by Brazil (more than 12 tons), Malaysia (153 kg) and the Netherlands (126 kg). Afghanistan reported having seized a total of 656 kg of paracetamol, in a number of instances.

180. With regard to cocaine, it is increasingly frequent for the cutting agents to be added directly to cocaine hydrochloride during the crystallization process in accordance with traffickers' requests. The substances reported in 2015 included benzocaine, lidocaine, mannitol and phenacetin; Colombia did not report the seizure of any cutting agents or diluents although the practice is known to occur there as well. **INCB encourages Governments to consider using information on cutting agents to trace the laboratories in which drugs are illicitly manufactured. Governments may also consider taking action against cutting agents in accordance with article 13 of the 1988 Convention.**

---

[28] National Narcotics Control Commission of China, *Annual Report on Drug Control in China 2016*.

IV. Prevention of chemical diversion beyond regulatory controls: the role of law enforcement

181. In its 2014 report on precursors, INCB provided a critical review and a strategic outlook of precursor control as a shared responsibility.[29] At that time, INCB identified preventive actions (in the form of industry cooperation and domestic controls) and law enforcement actions (stopping or seizing shipments of chemicals destined for illicit purposes) as central components of precursor control strategies that would be fit for the future. In its 2015 report on precursors, INCB elaborated on the merits and potential of public-private partnerships in preventing the diversion of chemicals. The present chapter aims at exploring the role of law enforcement actions in chemical diversion prevention and its interaction with regulatory controls.

Legal framework

182. The concept of precursor control as a complementary element of international drug control efforts was introduced some 25 years ago, by article 12 of the 1988 Convention. Because the substances that can be used in illicit drug manufacture have legitimate uses and are traded extensively and legitimately for those purposes, trade monitoring is the centrepiece of the international precursor control system.

183. In terms of law enforcement action, the 1988 Convention requires Governments to provide for the seizure of any substance in Table I or Table II if there is sufficient evidence that it is for use in the illicit manufacture of a narcotic drug or psychotropic substance (art. 12, para. 9 (b)). Governments are also obliged to provide INCB annually with the aggregated amounts of the seized substances and their origin, when known; information on any substance not included in Table I or II that has been identified as having been used or as being intended for use in the illicit manufacture of drugs or precursors; and information on methods of diversion and illicit manufacture (art. 12, para. 12).

184. For Governments to be able to comply with those obligations, they must be in a position to gather and consolidate the relevant information at the national level and hence have in place domestic legislation that provides for the seizure of substances listed in Tables I and II of the 1988 Convention as well as of substances not included in those tables when there is evidence that they are intended for use in illicit drug manufacture. In order to be able to have a comprehensive national situation report, Governments must also have in place a mechanism that enables full cooperation and information-sharing between all agencies responsible for precursor control. There is, however, a lack of national cooperation and coordination in many countries. In order to be effective, Governments must also be committed to precursor control in its entirety, that is, including not only regulatory elements but also law enforcement and investigative components. And, for the latter components to be effective, Governments must provide their enforcement authorities with the legal framework to take appropriate action, including the seizure of chemicals.

185. The international framework to establish a number of activities as criminal offences under domestic law is provided for in article 3, paragraph 1, of the 1988 Convention. With regard to chemical diversion control, the establishment of offences of manufacture, transport or distribution, knowing that they are to be used for illicit purposes, is mandatory on all parties (art. 3, para. 1 (a)(iv)), while the Convention leaves some latitude for the criminalization of mere possession of listed precursors (art. 3, para. 1 (c)(ii)).[30] In both cases, the Convention does not only refer to substances listed in Tables I and II but covers also equipment and materials. The provisions to establish criminal offences in article 3 therefore form a counterpart to the regulatory provisions of articles 12 and 13.

186. Nevertheless, INCB has noted that national authorities are looking for guidance, especially to address chemicals not under international control ("non-scheduled chemicals"). INCB has therefore compiled the provisions of the 1988 Convention that may be applied to address non-scheduled and substitute chemicals as part of its information package on the control of precursors, which is available for competent national authorities at the INCB secure web page. The compilation also includes the complementary measures requested by relevant resolutions of the Commission on Narcotic Drugs, the Economic and Social Council and the General Assembly.

---

[29] E/INCB/2014/4, paras. 7-35.

[30] The 1988 Convention also provides for the criminalization of the organization, management or financing of any of these offences, and to participation in, association or conspiracy to commit, attempts to commit, and facilitating the commission of any of the offences established in accordance with article 3 (art. 3, para. 1 (a)(v) and (c)(iv)).

Precursor law enforcement in practice

187. When a proposed shipment (through PEN Online) or actual shipment of precursors is suspended or stopped, a diversion attempt is discovered, a seizure is made, or an illicit laboratory is dismantled, the collection and timely dissemination of all information collected and intelligence generated, is critical. This will prepare the grounds for an effective follow-up investigation. The goal of such an investigation is to determine the source of the diverted precursors, the point and method of diversion, the method and route of transport and the criminal organizations involved in those activities. Competent national authorities are then in a position to shut down the particular route or method and prevent similar diversion attempts in the future. When the findings about diversions and attempted diversions are shared globally, alerting authorities worldwide, it helps to prevent future diversions that use the same or similar modus operandi.

188. Seizures of precursors, the stopping of shipments and the identification of cases of diversions and attempted diversions are therefore the beginning of a process — not the end. While seizure and other statistics may be a reflection of the level of law enforcement or regulatory activity and help to prevent a particular consignment of chemicals from reaching illicit laboratories, only complete and prompt follow-up investigations which lead to the discovery of relevant information will provide the means to address the gaps and weaknesses in control systems which, when closed, will ensure the long-lasting denial to traffickers of the chemicals they require.

189. The timely sharing of information on any chemical that is suspected of being used or that has actually been used in illicit drug manufacture, or information on attempts to divert a chemical into illicit channels, is critical to understanding, and addressing, new developments in the diversion of precursor chemicals and their use in illicit drug manufacture.

190. The systematic sharing of intelligence about seizures or suspected transactions also helps to build up evidence on the sources of supply and the methods of diversion of non-scheduled chemicals. This in turn enables the authorities of the alleged source countries to take action in the spirit of shared responsibility.[31] Significant reductions in seizures at Mexican and Central American ports of non-scheduled derivatives of phenylacetic acid, which can be used as pre-precursors of P-2-P (see Operation Phenylacetic Acid and its Derivatives (Operation PAAD), para. 194, below) and of methylamine (see Operation MMA, para. 194, below), provide evidence of the effectiveness of measures taken to limit exports of these chemicals to risk countries.

191. Diversion may happen at all stages of the distribution chain. Chemical diversion may affect all countries in which chemicals are manufactured, exported, imported, transited and used.

192. There is a shared responsibility to ensure that each and every national precursor control system is fit for its purpose and does not present a target for traffickers. There is also a need for full cooperation and willingness to investigate and share the results of law enforcement activity so as to develop a case and eventually identify the point of diversion, bring to justice those behind the diversion and prevent future diversions. Above all, the ultimate goal of precursor control remains effective diversion prevention, whereas seizures are, in fact, only indicators of known diversions that have been successful.

Role of the International Narcotics Control Board

193. To advance the law enforcement component of chemical diversion control in a practical manner, INCB has gathered focal points from 134 countries under Project Prism (focusing on synthetic drug precursors) and from 92 countries under Project Cohesion (focusing on precursors of cocaine and heroin). The two projects are steered by the Precursors Task Force with a view to soliciting direct, practical collaboration among nominated focal points, on an ongoing, ad hoc basis, on specific precursor aspects for limited periods of time, that is, during time-bound operations.

194. Recent Project Prism and Project Cohesion activities have helped to shed light on the use of a number of non-scheduled chemicals in illicit drug manufacture. These activities included a survey of the types of non-scheduled chemicals used for illicit drug manufacture (in 2014), and two operations focusing on esters and other non-scheduled derivatives of phenylacetic acid (Operation PAAD, in 2011) and on methylamine (Operation MMA, in 2015). Two additional operations focused on intelligence gaps in Africa with respect to ephedrine and pseudoephedrine (Operation Ephedrine and Pseudoephedrine Intelligence Gaps in Africa (Operation EPIG), in 2012) and on intelligence gaps related to acetic anhydride and glacial acetic acid, a

---

[31] Often, the chemical in question and the drug manufactured illicitly from it do not affect the source country's domestic market, and any action to prevent those chemicals from reaching clandestine laboratories elsewhere is therefore taken in the spirit of shared responsibility.

chemical that may be used to disguise smuggled acetic anhydride (Operation Eagle Eye, in 2013 and 2014).

195. Operation Eagle Eye was conducted in two phases: the first phase was collecting information on domestic movements of acetic anhydride and reviewing the legitimacy of domestic commerce in, and end use of, the substance, as well as the bona fides of companies involved, with a view to developing dedicated risk profiles; the second phase consisted of the identification and interdiction of trafficking of acetic anhydride to Afghanistan, inter alia, through the application of the risk profiles developed in the first phase.

196. It is clear from the above-mentioned examples that regulatory controls and trade monitoring cannot be separated from law enforcement action, as one feeds, and benefits from, the other. Precursor control is therefore a continuum which begins with a proper understanding of the legitimate market and the operators in that market, and up-to-date knowledge of trafficking trends and modi operandi, and which extends to the effective use of backtracking investigations, controlled or monitored deliveries, financial investigations, and other enforcement tools. Central to all this is the collection, sharing and utilization of intelligence. The Precursors Task Force, through INCB, operates as the global focal point for the exchange of such information and the coordination of international operational activities that cut across regulatory and law enforcement components of precursor control.

197. Cooperation with industry plays a critical role in the early identification of suspicious inquiries, orders and transactions based on unusual trade patterns or patterns incompatible with the inquirer's business model. The information from such industry alerts, when it is collated at the global level, can help to establish new global trends for the chemicals, including non-scheduled chemicals, in the focus of traffickers at a given time. That information subsequently feeds back into the work of national law enforcement authorities. More than 99.9 per cent of trade in chemicals is legitimate, and a suspicious inquiry may constitute an important piece of intelligence that can help to prevent a chemical from being used in illicit drug manufacture, even if there is not yet any criminal activity involved at that stage.

198. The participants in Project Prism and Project Cohesion also benefit from regular alerts that draw attention to diversion cases or new developments in terms of substances, modi operandi or trafficking trends, including companies involved in suspicious or illicit transactions. INCB facilitates the exchange of such intelligence at the global level, taking the necessary precautions to ensure there is no inappropriate condemnation of industries or countries that may have been the target of traffickers.

199. Since its launch in March 2012, PICS has become an important tool for participating Governments to communicate precursor information in real time with a view to launching joint investigations. As it is able to register users from multiple agencies, PICS also contributes to enhancing inter-agency communication at the national level. INCB also facilitates precursor case meetings between representatives of the countries concerned in order to aid intelligence-sharing and cooperation in backtracking investigations.

200. Based on information available, INCB facilitates international operational cooperation and shares strategic findings globally. This also includes information on legitimate uses, estimated annual legitimate requirements, non-scheduled substances that have been used in illicit manufacture of drugs or precursors, and information gained from stopped shipments and on thefts.

V. Conclusions

201. The present chapter contains broad conclusions and recommendations to address challenges to, and existing gaps in, the international precursor control system that have implications at the global level. A summary of the more detailed, technical recommendations, a number of which have already been made in previous years and are still valid, is available at the Board's website (www.incb.org).

Levels of international cooperation, communication and information-sharing between Governments and with INCB and the Precursors Task Force

202. Communication with some Governments remains problematic. In some cases, contact information for competent national authorities has never been provided or is outdated, inquiries about potentially suspicious transactions or seizures go unanswered, and the rate of participation and information exchange with INCB and the Precursors Task Force is insufficient. However, there are also encouraging examples of communication, such as when the liaison officers of Task Force members actively engage with the authorities of their host countries in the framework of Project Prism and Project Cohesion. INCB commends such efforts and encourages all Governments to improve operational cooperation at all levels. INCB also wishes to call on the Precursors Task Force members that are representatives of relevant international and regional organizations, such as

INTERPOL, the World Customs Organization and the Inter-American Drug Abuse Control Commission, to re-engage their members in international precursor control activities under Project Prism and Project Cohesion.

203. The level of detail of information shared about precursor seizures is generally low, which affects not only operational intervention but also INCB analysis of global and regional trends of the chemicals actually being used in illicit drug manufacture, their sources, the diversion methods and modi operandi of traffickers, as well as the dynamics of and interlinks between substances in Tables I and II of the 1988 Convention, substances in the limited international special surveillance list, and any non-scheduled substitutes or alternate chemicals.

204. In a number of recent cases, authorities of countries mentioned in PICS incidents have contacted the information provider, or INCB, to obtain further details in order to allow them to initiate investigations in their countries. Because many precursor seizures have an international dimension beyond the country in which the seizure occurred, any piece of information about the seizure is important as it could be the starting point of an investigation into the source of the chemical and the method of diversion. Governments are therefore encouraged to share all potentially actionable information through PICS or bilaterally, in the framework of Project Prism and Project Cohesion.[32]

Operation of the PEN Online system

205. As INCB has previously pointed out, the monitoring of international trade in scheduled substances has played a major role in limiting traffickers' access to those chemicals for illicit purposes. However, there continue to be loopholes, including the fact that some exporting countries do not use PEN Online to notify of exports or do not use the system systematically for all exports.[33]

206. More significantly, a further loophole is posed by the fact the authorities of a number of importing countries and territories which are registered to use PEN Online do not actually review incoming pre-export notifications. As a result, the authorities of the exporting countries are not in a position to determine whether the importing Government is aware of a planned shipment to its territory and has no objection, or whether it is unaware of the shipment and even unaware of the pre-export notification. This leaves the decision of whether or not a shipment should be authorized solely to the authority of the exporting country, and the importing country is at risk of being the target of traffickers' diversion attempts.

Integrity of controls on a Government's territory

207. Another issue of concern are territories where conflict, unresolved territorial disputes or other circumstances hinder the exercise of effective governmental control. Such territories are being exploited by traffickers who seek to divert precursor chemicals taking advantage of the vacuum of control.

208. To address some of those concerns, the INCB Precursors Task Force launched Operation Missing Links in October 2016, which seeks to close intelligence gaps with regard to the movement of precursors of methamphetamine and amphetamine (the active ingredient in fake "captagon" tablets) focusing on North Africa and the Middle East. Although the final results were not available at the time of writing this report, the authorities of some countries communicated major incidents involving amphetamine precursors, including in the preparatory phase of the operation that, for the first time, shed some light on the modi operandi of the illicit manufacturers and traffickers of "captagon".

209. An increasing number of proposed exports of precursor chemicals is destined for territories whose status is unclear, contested, or, at any given time, not effectively within the scope of control of an internationally recognized entity's competent national authorities. In these cases, exporting authorities will often be unable to pre-notify exports to an officially recognized counterpart, who has both the legal authority and the de facto capacity to provide adequate oversight and assurance regarding a shipment's end-purpose or destination. In such areas, there is a substantially increased risk of diversion of chemicals. In order to ensure the availability of controlled chemicals for legitimate purposes in all regions of the world, irrespective of a territory's status, and to manage associated risks, **INCB invites all Governments to work with the Board to devise appropriate ways and means of handling pre-export notifications in such cases with a view to enabling the trade of chemicals to and from high-risk areas in a regulated manner.**

---

[32] PICS does not provide for the sharing of nominal data. However, it is encouraged that it be indicated whether such data are available.

[33] This also includes consignments in the context of international missions, which are often sent without the knowledge, let alone the authorization, of the receiving Government.

210. Additionally, a frequent lack of sufficient transparency has previously been identified in connection with free trade zones and free ports. States parties are reminded that pursuant to article 18 of the 1988 Convention, they are obliged to apply control measures in free trade zones and free ports that are no less stringent than those applied in other parts of their territories.

National capacity to regulate precursors, monitor their trade and distribution and investigate precursor incidents

211. Insufficient attention to precursors matters within some government authorities may be due to limited national regulatory and enforcement capacity and, often, a lack of institutional memory due to considerable turnover of responsible staff. The lack of capacity is particularly apparent with regard to precursor investigations and in relation to the contributions that customs authorities could make in determining the modi operandi used by traffickers, in establishing suitable risk indicators for cross-border precursor trafficking and, ultimately, in generating actionable intelligence.

212. INCB has convened a workshop to that end in August 2016, with a focus on acetic anhydride and countries in West Asia. Chapter IV of the present report also reviews the law enforcement aspect of precursor control in detail, highlighting the growing importance of precursor investigations as the complexity of diversion patterns is increasing, and the value of such investigations as a preventive measure.

213. A framework for international operational cooperation in precursor matters is available, through the mechanisms and operations under Project Prism and Project Cohesion, and through PICS. Both, the thirtieth special session of the General Assembly on the world drug problem of April 2016, in its outcome document, and the Commission on Narcotic Drugs, in its resolution 59/8 of 22 March 2016, recognized the existing framework and encouraged Governments, in accordance with their national legislation, to make full use of the existing tools in order to address the sourcing and movement of, and trafficking in, scheduled and non-scheduled precursors.

The way forward

214. INCB invites all Governments and international and regional organizations to work with each other and the Board towards these goals, giving adequate attention to both regulatory and law enforcement aspects of precursor control, including customs-risk profiling, as well as partnerships with relevant sectors of industry as highlighted in the INCB report on precursors for 2015.

215. The present report has a special focus on the enforcement component of precursor control, which is becoming increasingly important because diversions of internationally controlled precursor chemicals from legitimate international trade are detected far less frequently than in the past, trafficking patterns are more complex, often involving domestic diversions with subsequent smuggling across international borders, and licit chemical markets are becoming increasingly diverse, not the least because of an increase in Internet-facilitated trade.

216. Changes in relation to the markets and patterns of trade of substances in Tables I and II are compounded by the emergence of non-scheduled chemicals, including series of related "designer" chemicals and chemicals made on demand, most of which are without legitimate use and/or trade.

217. A balanced mixture of enforcement and regulatory measures is therefore essential. What that right balance is can vary from one country to the next and depend on the particular substance, but the ultimate goal of all efforts must be to deny traffickers the chemicals they require to manufacture substances of abuse, and to cooperate to that end.

218. At present, however, precursors are often not a law enforcement priority. Significant amounts of critical information remain unnoticed or underutilized, and international law enforcement cooperation with respect to precursors is too often hampered by compartmentalization and lengthy or non-existent cooperation procedures. Far too often seizures are considered to be the end result of a law enforcement intervention. Available tools such as backtracking investigations or controlled (monitored) deliveries to identify and disrupt the sources and the criminal groups behind diversions are underutilized.

219. An increasingly large, complex, diversified and rapidly changing market for chemicals challenges authorities to devise solutions that allow for flexibility in enforcement interventions without adding the regulatory burden in the form of systematic international trade monitoring associated with the scheduling of a substance. While adding chemicals to the tables of the 1988 Convention will continue to be important for those chemicals most necessary for illicit drug manufacture, it is clear that effectively denying traffickers access to chemicals will also require active international cooperation on non-scheduled chemicals.

220. INCB has previously advocated that innovative solutions be implemented or tested in some countries, including the application of concepts such as that known as "immediate precursors" and the reversal of the burden of proof for suspicious transactions and stopped or suspended shipments. However, central to all these approaches is a legal framework which makes the supply[34] of any chemical for illicit purposes a crime, thus enabling law enforcement authorities to take action, exchange intelligence and cooperate across borders.

221. Article 12 of the 1988 Convention and relevant resolutions provide the fundamental framework for international cooperation to prevent chemicals from reaching clandestine laboratories and, subsequently, preventing illicitly manufactured drugs and new psychoactive substances from reaching consumer markets. INCB therefore considers precursor control to be an effective form of prevention of serious illicit activity, which deserves to be given much higher priority by Governments. INCB invites all Governments to cooperate and participate in the Board's initiatives to this end.

---

[34] Supply in this context refers to actions that lead to chemicals being available for illicit purposes (manufacture, acquisition and trafficking).

Glossary

The following terms and definitions have been used in the present report:

diversion:	Transfer of substances from licit to illicit channels
industrial-scale illicit laboratory:	Laboratory manufacturing synthetic drugs that uses oversized equipment and/or glassware that is either custom-made or purchased from industrial processing sources and/or that uses serial reactions; produces significant amounts of drugs in very short periods of time, the amount being limited only by the need for access to precursors and other essential chemicals in adequate quantities and for the logistics and manpower to handle large amounts of drugs and chemicals
monitored delivery:	A technique similar to a controlled delivery but which can occur in countries where no national legislation exists for controlled deliveries, where the substance is not internationally controlled or in cases where agreement to take part in a controlled delivery could not be reached by all involved competent national authorities in the time frame allotted
pharmaceutical formulation:	Mixture, typically a solid, prior to its formulation into a finished dosage form, that contains precursors present in such a way that they can be used or recovered by readily applicable means
pharmaceutical preparation:	Preparation for therapeutic (human or veterinary) use in its finished dosage form that contains precursors present in such a way that they can be used or recovered by readily applicable means; may be presented in their retail packaging or in bulk
seizure:	Prohibiting the transfer, conversion, disposition or movement of property or assuming custody or control of property on the basis of an order issued by a court or a competent authority; may be temporary or permanent (i.e., confiscation); different national legal systems may use different terms
stopped shipment:	Shipment permanently withheld because there are reasonable grounds to believe that it may constitute an attempted diversion, as a result of administrative problems or because of other grounds for concern or suspicion
suspended shipment:	Shipment temporarily withheld because of administrative inconsistencies or other grounds for concern or suspicion, for which clarification of the veracity of the order and resolution of technical issues are required before the shipment may be released
suspicious order (or suspicious transaction):	Order (or transaction) of questionable, dishonest or unusual character or condition, for which there is reason to believe that a chemical, which is being ordered, imported or exported or is transiting, is destined for the illicit manufacture of narcotic drugs or psychotropic substances.

Annexes*

---

*The annexes are not included in the printed version of the present report but they are available in the CD-ROM version and in the version on the website of the International Narcotics Control Board (www.incb.org).

Annex I

Parties and non-parties to the 1988 Convention, by region, as at 1 November 2016

Note: The date on which the instrument of ratification or accession was deposited is indicated in parentheses.

Region	Parties to the 1988 Convention		Non-parties to the 1988 Convention
Africa	Algeria (9 May 1995)	Eritrea (30 January 2002)	Equatorial Guinea
	Angola (26 October 2005)	Ethiopia (11 October 1994)	Somalia
	Benin (23 May 1997)	Gabon (10 July 2006)	South Sudan
	Botswana (13 August 1996)	Gambia (23 April 1996)	
	Burkina Faso (2 June 1992)	Ghana (10 April 1990)	
	Burundi (18 February 1993)	Guinea (27 December 1990)	
	Cabo Verde (8 May 1995)	Guinea-Bissau (27 October 1995)	
	Cameroon (28 October 1991)	Kenya (19 October 1992)	
	Central African Republic (15 October 2001)	Lesotho (28 March 1995)	
	Chad (9 June 1995)	Liberia (16 September 2005)	
	Comoros (1 March 2000)	Libya (22 July 1996)	
	Congo (3 March 2004)	Madagascar (12 March 1991)	
	Côte d'Ivoire (25 November 1991)	Malawi (12 October 1995)	
	Democratic Republic of the Congo (28 October 2005)	Mali (31 October 1995)	
	Djibouti (22 February 2001)	Mauritania (1 July 1993)	
	Egypt (15 March 1991)	Mauritius (6 March 2001)	

PRECURSORS

Region	Parties to the 1988 Convention		Non-parties to the 1988 Convention
	Morocco (28 October 1992)	South Africa (14 December 1998)	
	Mozambique (8 June 1998)	Sudan (19 November 1993)	
	Namibia (6 March 2009)	Swaziland (8 October 1995)	
	Niger (10 November 1992)	Togo (1 August 1990)	
	Nigeria (1 November 1989)	Tunisia (20 September 1990)	
	Rwanda (13 May 2002)	Uganda (20 August 1990)	
	Sao Tome and Principe (20 June 1996)	United Republic of Tanzania (17 April 1996)	
	Senegal (27 November 1989)	Zambia (28 May 1993)	
	Seychelles (27 February 1992)	Zimbabwe (30 July 1993)	
	Sierra Leone (6 June 1994)		
Regional total **54**		**51**	**3**
Americas	Antigua and Barbuda (5 April 1993)	Chile (13 March 1990)	
	Argentina (10 June 1993)	Colombia (10 June 1994)	
	Bahamas (30 January 1989)	Costa Rica (8 February 1991)	
	Barbados (15 October 1992)	Cuba (12 June 1996)	
	Belize (24 July 1996)	Dominica (30 June 1993)	
	Bolivia (Plurinational State of) (20 August 1990)	Dominican Republic (21 September 1993)	
	Brazil (17 July 1991)	Ecuador (23 March 1990)	
	Canada (5 July 1990)	El Salvador (21 May 1993)	

Region	Parties to the 1988 Convention		Non-parties to the 1988 Convention
	Grenada (10 December 1990)	Peru (16 January 1992)	
	Guatemala (28 February 1991)	Saint Kitts and Nevis (19 April 1995)	
	Guyana (19 March 1993)	Saint Lucia (21 August 1995)	
	Haiti (18 September 1995)	Saint Vincent and the Grenadines (17 May 1994)	
	Honduras (11 December 1991)	Suriname (28 October 1992)	
	Jamaica (29 December 1995)	Trinidad and Tobago (17 February 1995)	
	Mexico (11 April 1990)	United States of America (20 February 1990)	
	Nicaragua (4 May 1990)	Uruguay (10 March 1995)	
	Panama (13 January 1994)	Venezuela (Bolivarian Republic of) (16 July 1991)	
	Paraguay (23 August 1990)		
Regional total 35		35	0
Asia	Afghanistan (14 February 1992)	Cambodia (2 April 2005)	State of Palestine
	Armenia (13 September 1993)	China (25 October 1989)	
	Azerbaijan (22 September 1993)	Democratic People's Republic of Korea (19 March 2007)	
	Bahrain (7 February 1990)	Georgia (8 January 1998)	
	Bangladesh (11 October 1990)	India (27 March 1990)	
	Bhutan (27 August 1990)	Indonesia (23 February 1999)	
	Brunei Darussalam (12 November 1993)	Iran (Islamic Republic of) (7 December 1992)	

Region	Parties to the 1988 Convention	Non-parties to the 1988 Convention
	Iraq (22 July 1998)	Philippines (7 June 1996)	
	Israel (20 March 2002)	Qatar (4 May 1990)	
	Japan (12 June 1992)	Republic of Korea (28 December 1998)	
	Jordan (16 April 1990)	Saudi Arabia (9 January 1992)	
	Kazakhstan (29 April 1997)	Singapore (23 October 1997)	
	Kuwait (3 November 2000)	Sri Lanka (6 June 1991)	
	Kyrgyzstan (7 October 1994)	Syrian Arab Republic (3 September 1991)	
	Lao People's Democratic Republic (1 October 2004)	Tajikistan (6 May 1996)	
	Lebanon (11 March 1996)	Thailand (3 May 2002)	
	Malaysia (11 May 1993)	Timor-Leste (3 June 2014)	
	Maldives (7 September 2000)	Turkey (2 April 1996)	
	Mongolia (25 June 2003)	Turkmenistan (21 February 1996)	
	Myanmar (11 June 1991)	United Arab Emirates (12 April 1990)	
	Nepal (24 July 1991)	Uzbekistan (24 August 1995)	
	Oman (15 March 1991)	Viet Nam (4 November 1997)	
	Pakistan (25 October 1991)	Yemen (25 March 1996)	
Regional total	47	46	1
Europe	Albania (27 July 2001)	Austria[a] (11 July 1997)	
	Andorra (23 July 1999)	Belarus (15 October 1990)	

Region	Parties to the 1988 Convention		Non-parties to the 1988 Convention
	Belgium[a] (25 October 1995)	Luxembourg[a] (29 April 1992)	
	Bosnia and Herzegovina (1 September 1993)	Malta[a] (28 February 1996)	
	Bulgaria[a] (24 September 1992)	Monaco (23 April 1991)	
	Croatia[a] (26 July 1993)	Montenegro (3 June 2006)	
	Cyprus[a] (25 May 1990)	Netherlands[a] (8 September 1993)	
	Czechia[a,b] (30 December 1993)	Norway (14 November 1994)	
	Denmark[a] (19 December 1991)	Poland[a] (26 May 1994)	
	Estonia[a] (12 July 2000)	Portugal[a] (3 December 1991)	
	Finland[a] (15 February 1994)	Republic of Moldova (15 February 1995)	
	France[a] (31 December 1990)	Romania[a] (21 January 1993)	
	Germany[a] (30 November 1993)	Russian Federation (17 December 1990)	
	Greece[a] (28 January 1992)	San Marino (10 October 2000)	
	Holy See (25 January 2012)	Serbia (3 January 1991)	
	Hungary[a] (15 November 1996)	Slovakia[a] (28 May 1993)	
	Iceland (2 September 1997)	Slovenia[a] (6 July 1992)	
	Ireland[a] (3 September 1996)	Spain[a] (13 August 1990)	
	Italy[a] (31 December 1990)	Sweden[a] (22 July 1991)	
	Latvia[a] (25 February 1994)	Switzerland (14 September 2005)	
	Liechtenstein (9 March 2007)	The former Yugoslav Republic of Macedonia (13 October 1993)	

Region	Parties to the 1988 Convention		Non-parties to the 1988 Convention
	Lithuania[a] (8 June 1998)	Ukraine (28 August 1991)	
	United Kingdom of Great Britain and Northern Ireland[a] (28 June 1991)	European Union[c] (31 December 1990)	
Regional total **46**		**46**	**0**
Oceania	Australia (16 November 1992)	New Zealand (16 December 1998)	Kiribati
	Cook Islands (22 February 2005)	Niue (16 July 2012)	Palau
	Fiji (25 March 1993)	Samoa (19 August 2005)	Papua New Guinea
	Marshall Islands (5 November 2010)	Tonga (29 April 1996)	Soloman Islands
	Micronesia (Federated States of) (6 July 2004)	Vanuatu (26 January 2006)	Tuvalu
	Nauru (12 July 2012)		
Regional total **16**		**11**	**5**
World total **198**		**189**	**9**

[a] State member of the European Union.

[b] Since 17 May 2016, "Czechia" has replaced "Czech Republic" as the short name used in the United Nations.

[c] Extent of competence: article 12.

Annex II

Annual legitimate requirements for ephedrine, pseudoephedrine, 3,4-methylenedioxyphenyl-2-propanone and 1-phenyl-2-propanone, substances frequently used in the manufacture of amphetamine-type stimulants

1. In its resolution 49/3, entitled "Strengthening systems for the control of precursor chemicals used in the manufacture of synthetic drugs", the Commission on Narcotic Drugs:

    (a) Requested Member States to provide to the International Narcotics Control Board annual estimates of their legitimate requirements for 3,4-methylenedioxyphenyl-2-propanone (3,4-MDP-2-P), pseudoephedrine, ephedrine and 1-phenyl-2-propanone (P-2-P) and, to the extent possible, estimated requirements for imports of preparations containing those substances that could be easily used or recovered by readily applicable means;

    (b) Requested the Board to provide those estimates to Member States in such a manner as to ensure that such information was used only for drug control purposes;

    (c) Invited Member States to report to the Board on the feasibility and usefulness of preparing, reporting and using estimates of legitimate requirements for the precursor chemicals and preparations referred to above in preventing diversion.

2. Pursuant to that resolution, the Board formally invited Governments to prepare estimates of their legitimate requirements for those substances. Those estimates, as reported by Governments, were published, for the first time, in March 2007.

3. The table below reflects the latest data reported by Governments on those four precursor chemicals (and their preparations, as relevant). It is expected that those data will provide the competent authorities of exporting countries with at least an indication of the legitimate requirements of importing countries, thus preventing diversion attempts. Governments are invited to review their requirements as published, amend them as necessary and inform the Board of any required change. The data are current as at 1 November 2016; for updates, see www.incb.org/incb/en/precursors/alrs.html.

PRECURSORS

Annual legitimate requirements as reported by Governments for imports of ephedrine, pseudoephedrine, 3,4-methylenedioxyphenyl-2-propanone, 1-phenyl-2-propanone and their preparations, as at 1 November 2016
(Kilograms)

Country or territory	Ephedrine	Ephedrine preparations	Pseudoephedrine	Pseudoephedrine preparations	3,4-MDP-2-P[a]	P-2-P[b]
Afghanistan	0	50	0	3 000	0	0
Albania	6	0	5	0	0	0
Algeria	20		17 000		0	1
Argentina	18	0	19 000	144	0	0
Armenia	0	0	0	0	0	0
Ascension Island	0	0	0	0	0	0
Australia	5	8	4 800	1 680	0	1
Austria	146	23	1	1	1	1
Azerbaijan	20		10		0	0
Bahrain	0	0			0	
Bangladesh	200		49 021		0	0
Barbados	200		200	58	0[c]	
Belarus	0	25	25	20	0	0
Belgium	300	100	9 000	8 000	0	5
Belize			P	P	0[c]	
Benin	2	1	8	55	0[c]	
Bhutan	0	0	0	0	0	0
Bolivia (Plurinational State of)	41	0	3 649	2 902	0	0
Bosnia and Herzegovina	25	1	1 502	1 201	1	1
Botswana	300				0[c]	
Brazil	900[d]	0	20 000[d]	0	0	0
Brunei Darussalam	0	2	0	113	0	0
Bulgaria	100	296	0	0	0	0
Burundi		5		15	0[c]	
Cabo Verde	0	1	0	0	0	0
Cambodia	200	50	300	900	0[c]	
Cameroon	25			1	0[c]	
Canada	5 000	5	25 000		0	1
Chile	38	0	6 715	175	0	0
China	60 000		200 000		0[c]	
China, Hong Kong SAR	3 050	0	8 255	0	0	0
China, Macao SAR	1	10	1	159	0	0
Christmas Island	0	0	0	1	0	0
Cocos (Keeling) Islands	0	0	0	0	0	0
Colombia	0[e]	0[f]	1 845[e]	P	0	0
Cook Islands	0	0	0	1	0	0
Costa Rica	0	0	734	172	0	0

Country or territory	Ephedrine	Ephedrine preparations	Pseudoephedrine	Pseudoephedrine preparations	3,4-MDP-2-P[a]	P-2-P[b]
Côte d'Ivoire	30	1	25	500	0	0
Croatia	30	1	1	1	10	5
Cuba	200			6	0[c]	
Curaçao	0		0		0	0
Cyprus	10	10	600	270	0	0
Czechia[g]	266	4	819	396	0	0
Democratic People's Republic of Korea	1 000	1 200	0	0	2	0
Democratic Republic of the Congo	300	10	720	900	0[c]	
Denmark					0	0
Dominican Republic	75	4	300	175	0	0
Ecuador	10	6	600	2 500	0	0
Egypt	4 500	0	55 000	2 500	0	0
El Salvador	P(6)[h]	P(10)[h]	P	P	0	0
Eritrea	0	0	0	0	0	0
Estonia	5	5	1	500	0	0
Ethiopia	1 000			100		
Falkland Islands (Malvinas)	0	1	0	1	0[c]	0
Faroe Islands	0	0	0	0	0	0
Finland	4	60	1	650	0[c]	1
France	3 500	10	22 000	500	0	0
Gambia	0	0	0	0	0	0
Georgia	5	25	2	15	0	0
Germany	200		2 000		1	8
Ghana	4 500	300	3 000	200	0	0
Greece	1 000		600		0	0
Greenland	0	0	0	0	0	0
Guatemala	0		P	P	0	0
Guinea	36				0[c]	
Guinea-Bissau	0	0	0	0	0	0
Guyana	120	61	120	24	0	0
Haiti	200	1	350	11	0	0
Honduras	P	P(1)[f]	P	P	0	0
Hungary	850	0	1	0	0	1 800
Iceland	0	0	0	0	0	0
India	410 983	112 729	43 004	193 801	0	0
Indonesia	13 000	0	52 000	6 200	0	0
Iran (Islamic Republic of)	2	1	17 000	1	1	1
Iraq	3 000	100	14 000	10 000	0	P[i]
Ireland	0	30	0	426	0	0
Israel	30	3	3 600	360	0[c]	

PRECURSORS

Country or territory	Ephedrine	Ephedrine preparations	Pseudoephedrine	Pseudoephedrine preparations	3,4-MDP-2-P[a]	P-2-P[b]
Italy	100	0	30 000	0	0	0
Jamaica	50	150	500	300	0	0
Japan	1 000		12 000		0[c]	
Jordan	750		25 000		0[c]	P
Kazakhstan	0		0		0	0
Kenya	1 200	5	1 200	950	0	
Kyrgyzstan	0	0	0	100	0	0
Lao People's Democratic Republic	0	0	1 000	130	0	0
Latvia	20	35	65	350	0	0
Lebanon	52	2	500	800	0	0
Lithuania	1	1	1	600	1	1
Luxembourg	1	0	0	0	0	0
Madagascar	142	2	0	132	0	0
Malawi	1 000				0[c]	
Malaysia	6	8	3 406	2 310	0	0
Maldives	0	0	0	0	0	0
Malta	0	220	0	220	0	0
Mauritius	0	0	0	0	0	0
Mexico	P(500)[h]	P[h]	P	P	0	0
Monaco	0	0	0	0	0	0
Mongolia	3				0[c]	
Montenegro	0	2	0	150	0	0
Montserrat	0	1	0	1	0	0
Morocco	41	15	2 929	0	0	0
Mozambique	3				0[c]	
Myanmar	2	11	0	0	0	0
Namibia	0	0	0	0	0	0
Nepal		1	5 000		0[c]	
Netherlands	1 200	50	500	0	0	0
New Zealand	50	0	1 000		0	3
Nicaragua	P[i]	P[i]	P	P	0	0
Nigeria	9 650	500	5 823	15 000	0	0
Norfolk Island	0	0	0	0	0	0
Norway	26	0	1	1	0	0
Oman	1		228		0[c]	
Pakistan	10 000		48 000	500	0[c]	
Panama	6	6	400	500	0	
Papua New Guinea	1		200		0	0
Paraguay	0	0	2 500	0	0	0
Peru	46	0	2 524	1 078	0	

Country or territory	Ephedrine	Ephedrine preparations	Pseudoephedrine	Pseudoephedrine preparations	3,4-MDP-2-P[a]	P-2-P[b]
Philippines	12	0	149	0	0	0
Poland	170	100	5 160	3 000	1	4
Portugal			15		0[c]	
Qatar	0	0	0	80	0	0
Republic of Korea	29 951		34 700		1	1
Republic of Moldova	0	0	0	600	0	0
Romania	135		2 424		0	0
Russian Federation	1 500				0[c]	
Rwanda		10		10	2	2
Saint Helena	0	1	0	1	0	0
Saint Lucia	0	6	0	15	0	0
Saint Vincent and the Grenadines	0		0		0	0
Sao Tome and Principe	0	0	0	0	0	0
Saudi Arabia	1	0	12 000	0	0	0
Senegal	82	1	0	510	0	0
Serbia	25	0	1 265	0	0	1
Singapore	8 910	6	52 385	2 387	1	1
Slovakia	4	6	1	1	0	0
Slovenia	6		250		0	0
Solomon Islands	0	1	0	1	0	0
South Africa	13 900	0	10 444	10 816	0	0
Spain	236		3 838		0	111
Sri Lanka		0		0	0	0
Sweden	186	167	2	1	1	11
Switzerland	2 600		80 000		1	500
Syrian Arab Republic	1 000		50 000		0[c]	
Tajikistan	38				0[c]	
Thailand	53	0	1	0	0	0
Trinidad and Tobago					0[c]	0
Tristan da Cunha	0	0	0	0	0	0
Tunisia	1	18	4 000	0	0	30
Turkey	200	0	26 500	5 000	0	0
Turkmenistan	0	0	0	0	0	0
Uganda	150	35	3 000	200	0	0
Ukraine	0	36	0	0	0	0
United Arab Emirates	0		3 000	2 499	0	0
United Kingdom	64 448	1 011	25 460	1 683	8	1
United Republic of Tanzania	100	1 500	2 000	100	0[c]	
United States of America	5 000		224 507		0[c]	41 740
Uruguay	0	0	1	0	0	0

Country or territory	Ephedrine	Ephedrine preparations	Pseudoephedrine	Pseudoephedrine preparations	3,4-MDP-2-P[a]	P-2-P[b]
Uzbekistan	0	0	0		0	0
Venezuela (Bolivarian Republic of)	60	0	2 425	0	0	0
Yemen	75	75	3 000	2 000	0[c]	
Zambia	50	25	50	100	0[c]	
Zimbabwe	150	1	150	50	0	0

Notes: The names of territories, departments and special administrative regions are in italics.

A blank field signifies that no requirement was indicated or that data were not submitted for the substance in question.

A zero (0) signifies that the country or territory currently has no licit requirement for the substance.

The letter "P" signifies that importation of the substance is prohibited.

Reported quantities of less than 1 kg have been rounded up and are reflected as 1 kg.

[a] 3,4-Methylenedioxyphenyl-2-propanone.

[b] 1-Phenyl-2-propanone.

[c] The Board is currently unaware of any legitimate need for the importation of this substance into the country.

[d] Including the legitimate requirements for pharmaceutical preparations containing the substance.

[e] The required amount of ephedrine is to be used for the manufacture of injectable ephedrine sulphate solution. The required amount of pseudoephedrine is to be used exclusively for the manufacture of medicines for export.

[f] In the form of injectable ephedrine sulphate solution.

[g] Since 17 May 2016, "Czechia" has replaced "Czech Republic" as the short name used in the United Nations.

[h] Imports of the substance and preparations containing the substance are prohibited, with the exception of the imports of injectable ephedrine preparations and ephedrine as a prime raw material for the manufacture of such ephedrine preparations. Pre-export notification is required for each individual import.

[i] Includes products containing P-2-P.

[j] Imports of the substance and preparations containing the substance are prohibited, with the exception of the imports of injectable ephedrine preparations and ephedrine as a prime raw material for the manufacture of such ephedrine preparations. Such export requires an import permit.

Annex III

Substances in Tables I and II of the 1988 Convention

Table I

Acetic anhydride
N-Acetylanthranilic acid
Ephedrine
Ergometrine
Ergotamine
Isosafrole
Lysergic acid
3,4-Methylenedioxyphenyl-2-propanone
Norephedrine
Phenylacetic acid
alpha-Phenylacetoacetonitrile[b]
1-Phenyl-2-propanone
Piperonal
Potassium permanganate
Pseudoephedrine
Safrole

The salts of the substances listed in this Table whenever the existence of such salts is possible.

Table II

Acetone
Anthranilic acid
Ethyl ether
Hydrochloric acid[a]
Methyl ethyl ketone
Piperidine
Sulphuric acid[a]
Toluene

The salts of the substances listed in this Table whenever the existence of such salts is possible.

[a] The salts of hydrochloric acid and sulphuric acid are specifically excluded from Table II.
[b] Included in Table I, effective 6 October 2014.

Annex IV

Use of scheduled substances in the illicit manufacture of narcotic drugs and psychotropic substances

Figures A.I-A.IV below depict the use of scheduled substances in the illicit manufacture of narcotic drugs and psychotropic substances. The approximate quantities provided are based on common manufacturing methods. Other manufacturing methods using scheduled substances — or even non-scheduled substances instead of or in addition to scheduled substances — may also be encountered, depending on the geographical location.

Figure A.I. Illicit manufacture of cocaine and heroin: scheduled substances and the approximate quantities thereof required for the illicit manufacture of 100 kilograms of cocaine or heroin hydrochloride

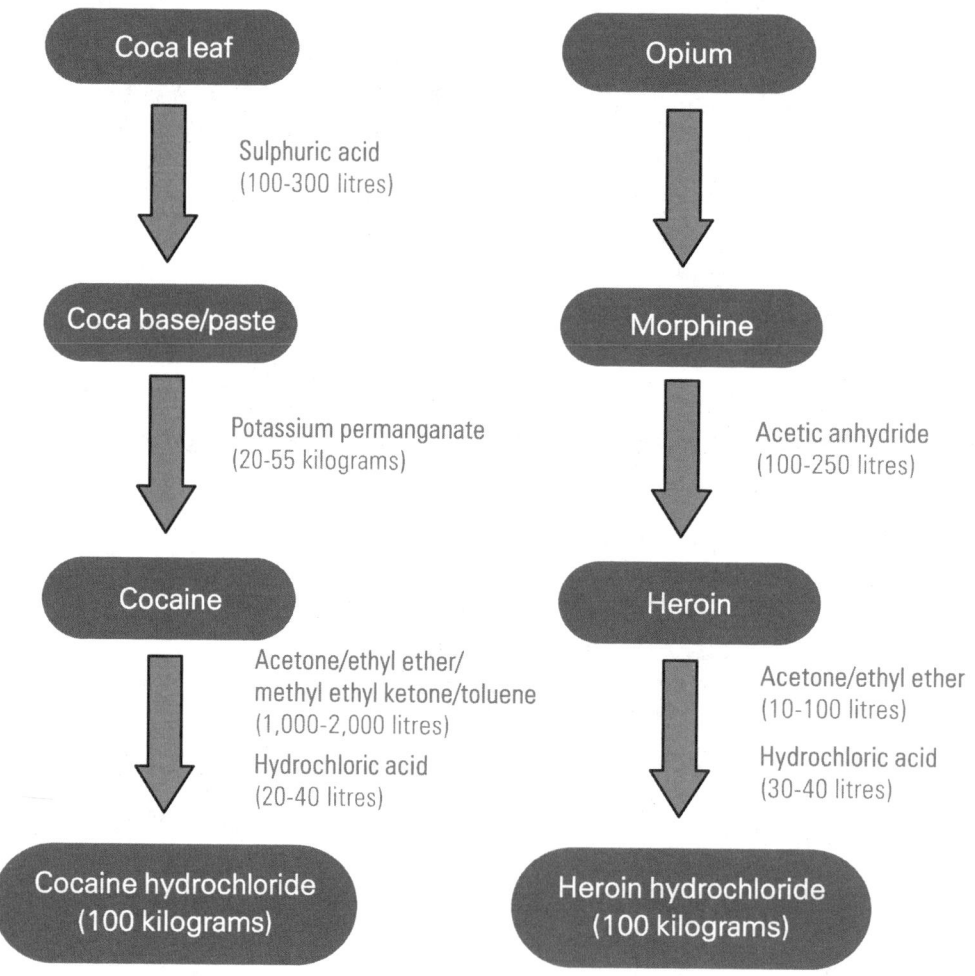

Note: The extraction of cocaine from coca leaf and the purification of coca paste and the crude base products of cocaine and heroin require solvents, acids and bases. A wide range of such chemicals have been used at all stages of drug manufacture.

Figure A.II. Illicit manufacture of amphetamine and methamphetamine: scheduled substances and the approximate quantities thereof required for the illicit manufacture of 100 kilograms of amphetamine sulphate and methamphetamine hydrochloride

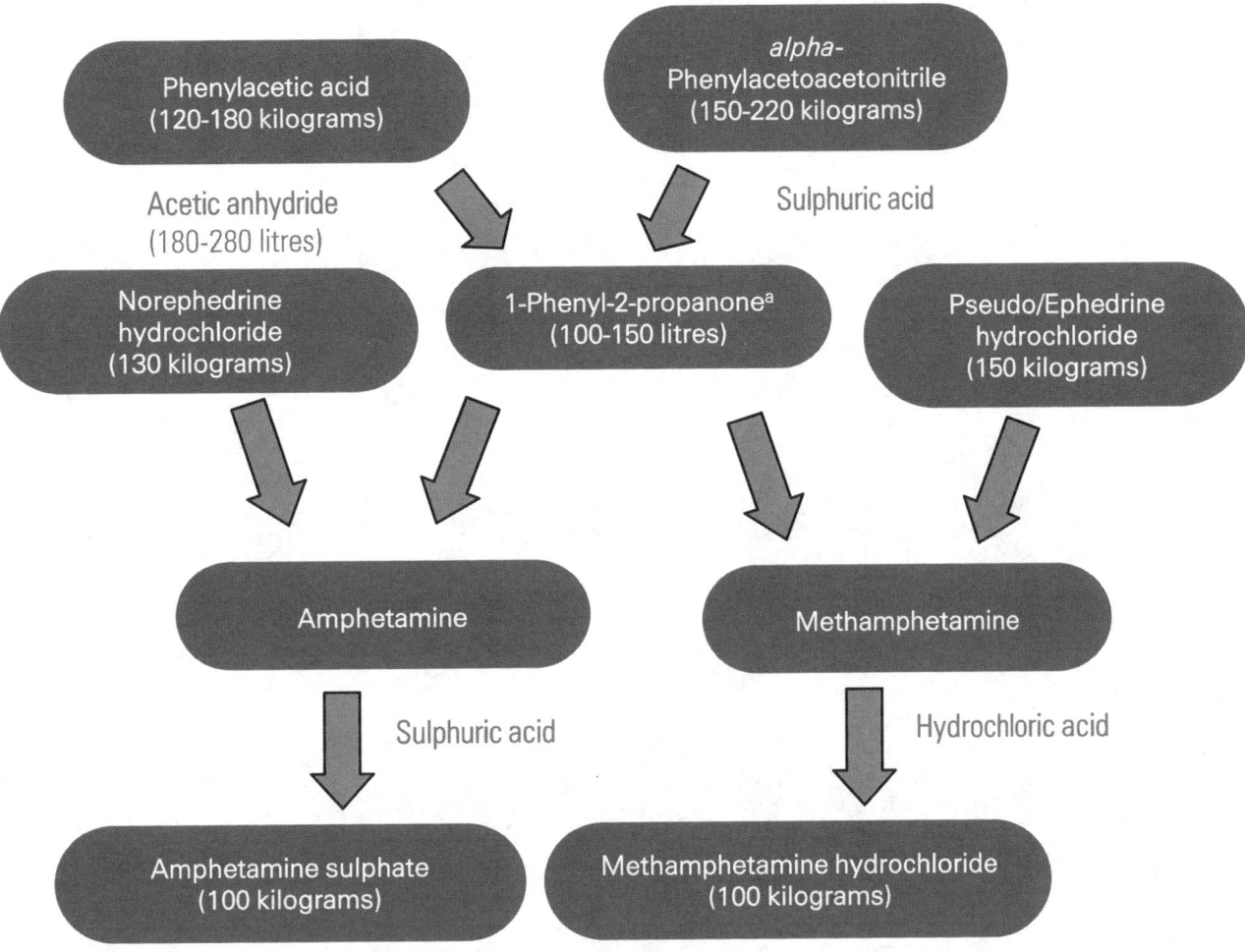

Note: Methcathinone, a less commonly encountered amphetamine-type stimulant, can be manufactured from pseudo/ephedrine hydrochloride, requiring the same approximate quantities as methamphetamine to yield 100 kilograms of hydrochloride salt.

[a] Methods based on 1-phenyl-2-propanone result in racemic *d,l*-meth/amphetamine while methods based on ephedrine, pseudoephedrine or norephedrine result in *d*-meth/amphetamine.

Figure A.III. Illicit manufacture of 3,4-methylenedioxymethamphetamine (MDMA) and related drugs: scheduled substances and the approximate quantities thereof required for the illicit manufacture of 100 kilograms of MDMA

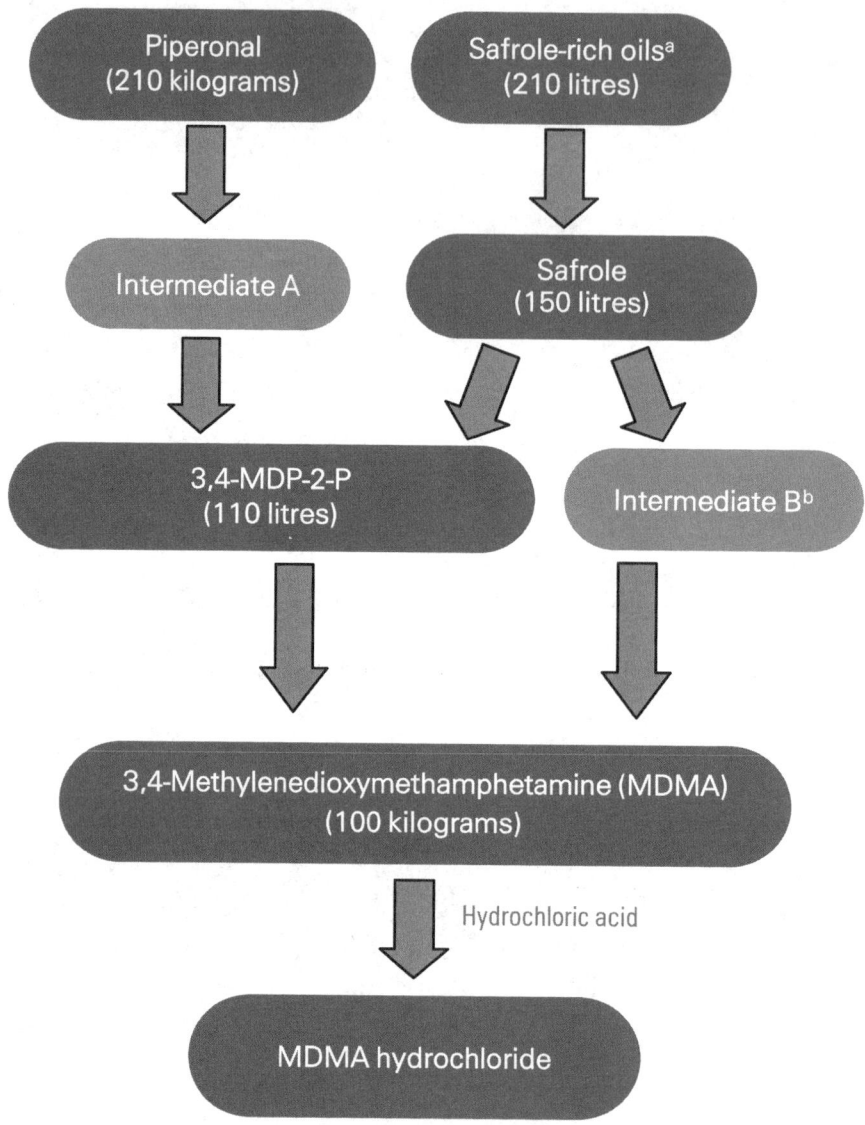

Note: Isosafrole, another precursor of MDMA under international control, is not included in this scheme, as it is not commonly encountered as a starting material; it is an intermediate in a modification of methods for manufacturing MDMA from safrole, requiring approximately 300 litres of safrole to manufacture 100 kilograms of MDMA.

[a] Assuming the safrole-rich oils have a safrole content of 75 per cent or higher.

[b] The manufacture of 100 kilograms of MDMA via intermediate B would require 200 litres of safrole.

Figure A.IV. Illicit manufacture of lysergic acid diethylamide (LSD), methaqualone and phencyclidine: scheduled substances and the approximate quantities thereof required for the illicit manufacture of 1 kilogram of LSD and 100 kilograms of methaqualone and phencyclidine

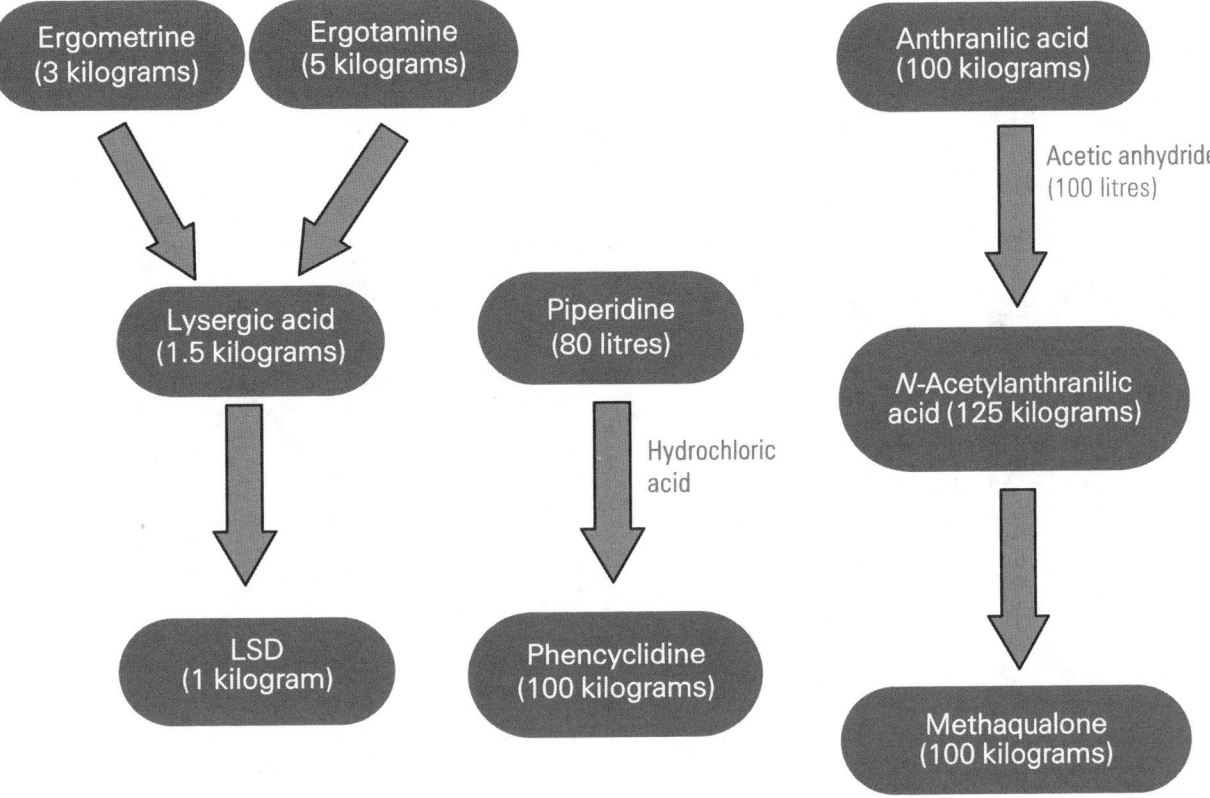

Annex V

Treaty provisions for the control of substances frequently used in the illicit manufacture of narcotic drugs and psychotropic substances

1. Article 2, paragraph 8, of the Single Convention on Narcotic Drugs of 1961 as amended by the 1972 Protocol[a] provides as follows:

> The Parties shall use their best endeavours to apply to substances which do not fall under this Convention, but which may be used in the illicit manufacture of drugs, such measures of supervision as may be practicable.

2. Article 2, paragraph 9, of the Convention on Psychotropic Substances of 1971[b] provides as follows:

> The Parties shall use their best endeavours to apply to substances which do not fall under this Convention, but which may be used in the illicit manufacture of psychotropic substances, such measures of supervision as may be practicable.

3. Article 12 of the United Nations Convention against Illicit Traffic in Narcotic Drugs and Psychotropic Substances of 1988[c] contains provisions for the following:

   (a) General obligation for parties to take measures to prevent diversion of the substances in Tables I and II of the 1988 Convention and to cooperate with each other to that end (para. 1);

   (b) Mechanism for amending the scope of control (paras. 2-7);

   (c) Requirement to take appropriate measures to monitor manufacture and distribution, to which end parties may control persons and enterprises, control establishments and premises under licence, require permits for such operations and prevent accumulation of substances in Tables I and II (para. 8);

   (d) Obligation to monitor international trade in order to identify suspicious transactions, to provide for seizures, to notify the authorities of the parties concerned in case of suspicious transactions, to require proper labelling and documentation and to ensure maintenance of such documents for at least two years (para. 9);

   (e) Mechanism for advance notice of exports of substances in Table I, upon request (para. 10);

   (f) Confidentiality of information (para. 11);

   (g) Reporting by parties to the International Narcotics Control Board (para. 12);

   (h) Report of the Board to the Commission on Narcotic Drugs (para. 13);

   (i) Non-applicability of the provisions of article 12 to certain preparations (para. 14).

---

[a] United Nations, *Treaty Series*, vol. 976, No. 14152.
[b] Ibid., vol. 1019, No. 14956.
[c] Ibid., vol. 1582, No. 27627.

Annex VI

Regional groupings

Reference is made throughout the present report to various geographical regions, which are defined as follows:

Africa: Algeria, Angola, Benin, Botswana, Burkina Faso, Burundi, Cabo Verde, Cameroon, Central African Republic, Chad, Comoros, Congo, Côte d'Ivoire, Democratic Republic of the Congo, Djibouti, Egypt, Equatorial Guinea, Eritrea, Ethiopia, Gabon, Gambia, Ghana, Guinea, Guinea-Bissau, Kenya, Lesotho, Liberia, Libya, Madagascar, Malawi, Mali, Mauritania, Mauritius, Morocco, Mozambique, Namibia, Niger, Nigeria, Rwanda, Sao Tome and Principe, Senegal, Seychelles, Sierra Leone, Somalia, South Africa, South Sudan, Sudan, Swaziland, Togo, Tunisia, Uganda, United Republic of Tanzania, Zambia and Zimbabwe;

Central America and the Caribbean: Antigua and Barbuda, Bahamas, Barbados, Belize, Costa Rica, Cuba, Dominica, Dominican Republic, El Salvador, Grenada, Guatemala, Haiti, Honduras, Jamaica, Nicaragua, Panama, Saint Kitts and Nevis, Saint Lucia, Saint Vincent and the Grenadines and Trinidad and Tobago;

North America: Canada, Mexico and United States of America;

South America: Argentina, Bolivia (Plurinational State of), Brazil, Chile, Colombia, Ecuador, Guyana, Paraguay, Peru, Suriname, Uruguay and Venezuela (Bolivarian Republic of);

East and South-East Asia: Brunei Darussalam, Cambodia, China, Democratic People's Republic of Korea, Indonesia, Japan, Lao People's Democratic Republic, Malaysia, Mongolia, Myanmar, Philippines, Republic of Korea, Singapore, Thailand, Timor-Leste and Viet Nam;

South Asia: Bangladesh, Bhutan, India, Maldives, Nepal and Sri Lanka;

West Asia: Afghanistan, Armenia, Azerbaijan, Bahrain, Georgia, Iran (Islamic Republic of), Iraq, Israel, Jordan, Kazakhstan, Kuwait, Kyrgyzstan, Lebanon, Oman, Pakistan, Qatar, Saudi Arabia, State of Palestine, Syrian Arab Republic, Tajikistan, Turkey, Turkmenistan, United Arab Emirates, Uzbekistan and Yemen;

Europe:

    Eastern Europe: Belarus, Republic of Moldova, Russian Federation and Ukraine;

    South-Eastern Europe: Albania, Bosnia and Herzegovina, Bulgaria, Croatia, Montenegro, Romania, Serbia and the former Yugoslav Republic of Macedonia;

    Western and Central Europe: Andorra, Austria, Belgium, Cyprus, Czechia[a] Republic, Denmark, Estonia, Finland, France, Germany, Greece, Holy See, Hungary, Iceland, Ireland, Italy, Latvia, Liechtenstein, Lithuania, Luxembourg, Malta, Monaco, Netherlands, Norway, Poland, Portugal, San Marino, Slovakia, Slovenia, Spain, Sweden, Switzerland and United Kingdom of Great Britain and Northern Ireland;

Oceania: Australia, Cook Islands, Fiji, Kiribati, Marshall Islands, Micronesia (Federated States of), Nauru, New Zealand, Niue, Palau, Papua New Guinea, Samoa, Solomon Islands, Tonga, Tuvalu and Vanuatu.

---

[a] Since 17 May 2016, "Czechia" has replaced "Czech Republic" as the short name used in the United Nations.

Annex VII

Submission of information by Governments pursuant to article 12 of the 1988 Convention (form D) for the years 2011-2015

Notes: The names of non-metropolitan territories and special administrative regions are in italics.
A blank signifies that form D was not received.
"X" signifies that a completed form D (or equivalent report) was submitted, including nil returns.
Entries for parties to the 1988 Convention (and for the years that they have been parties) are shaded.

Country or territory	2011	2012	2013	2014	2015
Afghanistan	X	X	X	X	X
Albania	X	X	X	X	X
Algeria	X	X	X	X	
Andorra	X	X	X	X	X
Angola					
Anguilla[a]			X		
Antigua and Barbuda					
Argentina	X	X	X	X	X
Armenia	X	X	X	X	X
Aruba[a]					
Ascension Island	X	X			
Australia	X	X	X	X	X
Austria[b]	X	X	X	X	X
Azerbaijan	X	X	X	X	X
Bahamas					
Bahrain				X	X
Bangladesh	X	X	X	X	X
Barbados			X		
Belarus	X	X	X	X	X
Belgium[b]	X	X	X	X	X
Belize			X		
Benin	X	X	X	X	X
Bermuda[a]					
Bhutan	X	X		X	X
Bolivia (Plurinational State of)	X	X	X	X	X
Bosnia and Herzegovina	X	X	X	X	X
Botswana					
Brazil	X	X	X	X	X
British Virgin Islands[a]					
Brunei Darussalam	X	X	X	X	X
Bulgaria	X	X	X	X	X
Burkina Faso	X				
Burundi					X
Cabo Verde					X
Cambodia	X	X	X	X	
Cameroon	X	X	X	X	
Canada	X	X	X	X	X
Cayman Islands[a]		X	X	X	
Central African Republic					

Country or territory	2011	2012	2013	2014	2015
Chad			X		
Chile	X	X	X	X	X
China	X	X	X	X	X
China, Hong Kong SAR		X	X		
China, Macao SAR		X	X	X	
Christmas Island[a,c]	X		X	X	X
Cocos (Keeling) Islands[a,c]	X		X	X	X
Colombia	X	X	X	X	X
Comoros					
Congo					
Cook Islands	X				
Costa Rica	X	X	X	X	X
Côte d'Ivoire	X	X	X	X	
Croatia[b]	X	X	X	X	X
Cuba	X				
Curaçao	X	X	X	X	X
Cyprus[b]	X	X	X	X	X
Czechia[b,d]	X	X	X	X	X
Democratic People's Republic of Korea	X	X	X		X
Democratic Republic of the Congo	X	X	X		X
Denmark[b]	X	X	X	X	X
Djibouti					
Dominica					
Dominican Republic			X	X	
Ecuador	X	X	X	X	X
Egypt	X	X	X	X	X
El Salvador	X	X	X	X	X
Equatorial Guinea					
Eritrea	X	X			
Estonia[b]	X	X	X	X	X
Ethiopia	X	X	X		X
Falkland Islands (Malvinas)	X	X	X	X	X
Fiji	X				
Finland[b]	X	X	X	X	X
France[b]	X	X	X	X	X
French Polynesia[a]					X
Gabon					
Gambia	X		X		
Georgia	X	X	X	X	X
Germany[b]	X	X	X	X	X
Ghana	X	X	X	X	X
Gibraltar					
Greece[b]	X	X	X	X	X
Grenada					
Guatemala	X	X	X	X	X
Guinea					
Guinea-Bissau		X			
Guyana				X	X
Haiti	X		X	X	X
Holy See[e]					

PRECURSORS

Country or territory	2011	2012	2013	2014	2015
Honduras	X	X	X		X
Hungary[b]	X	X	X	X	X
Iceland	X	X	X	X	X
India	X	X	X	X	X
Indonesia	X	X	X	X	X
Iran (Islamic Republic of)			X	X	X
Iraq	X				
Ireland[b]	X	X	X	X	X
Israel	X	X	X	X	X
Italy[b]	X	X	X	X	X
Jamaica			X	X	X
Japan	X	X	X	X	X
Jordan	X	X	X	X	X
Kazakhstan	X	X	X		X
Kenya					X
Kiribati					
Kuwait		X	X		
Kyrgyzstan	X	X	X	X	X
Lao People's Democratic Republic	X	X	X	X	X
Latvia[b]	X	X	X	X	X
Lebanon	X	X	X	X	X
Lesotho					
Liberia					
Libya					
Liechtenstein[f]					
Lithuania[b]	X	X	X	X	X
Luxembourg[b]	X	X	X	X	
Madagascar			X	X	X
Malawi					
Malaysia	X	X	X	X	X
Maldives	X	X	X		
Mali			X		X
Malta[b]	X	X	X	X	X
Marshall Islands					
Mauritania					
Mauritius	X	X			
Mexico	X	X	X	X	X
Micronesia (Federated States of)			X		
Monaco[g]					
Mongolia		X			X
Montenegro	X	X	X	X	X
Montserrat[a]		X	X	X	X
Morocco	X	X	X	X	X
Mozambique				X	
Myanmar	X	X	X	X	X
Namibia				X	
Nauru					
Nepal			X	X	
Netherlands[b]	X	X	X	X	X
New Caledonia[a]	X	X	X	X	X

Country or territory	2011	2012	2013	2014	2015
New Zealand	X	X	X		X
Nicaragua	X	X	X	X	X
Niger					
Nigeria	X	X	X		
Niue					
Norfolk Island[c]	X		X	X	X
Norway		X	X	X	X
Oman				X	X
Pakistan	X	X	X	X	X
Palau			X		
Panama	X	X	X	X	X
Papua New Guinea					
Paraguay	X		X		
Peru	X	X	X	X	X
Philippines	X	X	X	X	X
Poland[b]	X	X	X	X	X
Portugal[b]	X	X	X	X	X
Qatar	X		X		
Republic of Korea	X	X	X	X	X
Republic of Moldova	X	X	X	X	X
Romania[b]	X	X	X	X	X
Russian Federation	X	X	X	X	X
Rwanda					X
Saint Helena	X				
Saint Kitts and Nevis					
Saint Lucia	X	X	X	X	X
Saint Vincent and the Grenadines		X	X	X	X
Samoa	X	X			
San Marino[e]					
Sao Tome and Principe	X				
Saudi Arabia	X	X	X	X	X
Senegal			X	X	X
Serbia	X	X	X		
Seychelles	X	X			
Sierra Leone					
Singapore	X	X	X	X	X
Sint Maarten					
Slovakia[b]	X	X	X	X	X
Slovenia[b]	X	X	X	X	X
Solomon Islands					
Somalia					
South Africa			X		X
South Sudan					
Spain[b]	X	X	X	X	X
Sri Lanka	X	X	X	X	X
Sudan				X	X
Suriname					
Swaziland					
Sweden[b]	X	X	X	X	X
Switzerland	X	X	X	X	X

PRECURSORS

Country or territory	2011	2012	2013	2014	2015
Syrian Arab Republic		X	X	X	X
Tajikistan	X	X	X		X
Thailand	X	X	X	X	X
The former Yugoslav Republic of Macedonia					
Timor-Leste					
Togo		X			
Tonga					
Trinidad and Tobago	X	X	X	X	X
Tristan da Cunha					
Tunisia	X	X	X	X	X
Turkey	X	X	X	X	X
Turkmenistan	X	X	X	X	X
Turks and Caicos Islands[a]					
Tuvalu	X	X			
Uganda	X	X	X	X	X
Ukraine	X	X	X		X
United Arab Emirates	X	X	X	X	X
United Kingdom[b]	X	X	X	X	X
United Republic of Tanzania	X	X	X	X	X
United States of America	X	X	X	X	X
Uruguay	X	X	X	X	X
Uzbekistan	X	X	X	X	X
Vanuatu	X				
Venezuela (Bolivarian Republic of)	X	X	X	X	X
Viet Nam	X	X	X	X	X
Wallis and Futuna Islands[a]					
Yemen	X	X			
Zambia				X	
Zimbabwe			X	X	X
Total number of governments that submitted form D	134	130	141	127	129
Total number of governments requested to provide information	213	213	213	213	213

[a] Territorial application of the 1988 Convention has been confirmed by the authorities concerned.
[b] State member of the European Union.
[c] Information was provided by Australia.
[d] Since 17 May 2016, "Czechia" has replaced "Czech Republic" as the short name used in the United Nations.
[e] The Holy See and San Marino did not furnish form D separately as their data are included in the report of Italy.
[f] Liechtenstein did not furnish form D separately as its data are included in the report of Switzerland.
[g] Monaco did not furnish form D separately as its data are included in the report of France.

Annex VIII

Seizures of substances in Tables I and II of the 1988 Convention, as reported to the International Narcotics Control Board, 2011-2015

1. Tables A.1 and A.2 below show information on seizures of the substances included in Tables I and II of the United Nations Convention against Illicit Traffic in Narcotic Drugs and Psychotropic Substances of 1988, furnished to the International Narcotics Control Board by Governments in accordance with article 12, paragraph 12, of the Convention.

2. The tables include data on domestic seizures and on seizures effected at points of entry or exit. They do not include reported seizures of substances where it is known that the substances were not intended for the illicit manufacture of drugs (for example, seizures effected on administrative grounds or seizures of ephedrine/pseudoephedrine preparations to be used as stimulants). Stopped shipments are also not included. The information may include data submitted by Governments through means other than form D; in such cases, the sources are duly noted.

Units of measure and conversion factors

3. Units of measure are indicated for every substance. As fractions of full units are not listed in the tables, figures are rounded as necessary.

4. For a variety of reasons, individual quantities of some substances seized are reported to the Board using different units; for instance, one country may report seizures of acetic anhydride in litres, another in kilograms.

5. To enable a proper comparison of collected information, it is important that all data be collated in a standard format. To simplify the necessary standardization process, figures are given in grams or kilograms where the substance is a solid and in litres where the substance (or its most common form) is a liquid.

6. Seizures of solids reported to the Board in litres have not been converted into kilograms and are not included in the tables, as the actual quantity of substance in solution is not known.

7. For seizures of liquids, quantities reported in kilograms have been converted into litres using the following factors:

Substance	Conversion factor (kilograms to litres)[a]
Acetic anhydride	0.926
Acetone	1.269
Ethyl ether	1.408
Hydrochloric acid (39.1% solution)	0.833
Isosafrole	0.892
3,4-Methylenedioxyphenyl-2-propanone	0.833
Methyl ethyl ketone	1.242

[a] Derived from density (The Merck Index (Rahway, New Jersey, Merck, 1989)).

1-Phenyl-2-propanone	0.985
Piperidine	1.160
Safrole	0.912
Sulphuric acid (concentrated solution)	0.543
Toluene	1.155

8. As an example, to convert 1,000 kilograms of methyl ethyl ketone into litres, multiply by 1.242, i.e. 1,000 × 1.242 = 1,242 litres.

9. For the conversion of gallons to litres, it has been assumed that in Colombia the United States gallon is used, with 3.785 litres to the gallon, and in Myanmar the imperial gallon is used, with 4.546 litres to the gallon.

10. If reported quantities have been converted, the converted figures are listed in the tables in italics.

11. The names of territories appear in italics.

12. A dash (–) signifies that the report did not include data on seizures of the particular substance in the reporting year.

13. A degree symbol (°) signifies less than the smallest unit of measurement shown for that substance (for example, less than 1 kilogram).

14. Discrepancies may exist between the regional total seizure figures and the world total figures because the actual quantities seized were rounded to whole numbers.

Table A.1. Seizures of substances in Tables I and II of the 1988 Convention as reported to the International Narcotics Control Board, 2011-2015

Country / Year	Acetic anhydride (litres)	N-Acetylanthranilic acid (kilograms)	Ephedrine (kilograms)	Ephedrine preparations[a] (kilograms)	Ergometrine (grams)	Ergotamine (grams)	Isosafrole (litres)	Lysergic acid (grams)	3,4-Methylenedioxyphenyl-2-propanone (litres)	Norephedrine (phenylpropanolamine) (kilograms)	Phenylacetic acid (kilograms)	alpha-phenylacetoacetonitrile (APAAN)[b] (kilograms)	1-Phenyl-2-propanone (litres)	Piperonal (kilograms)	Potassium permanganate (kilograms)	Pseudoephedrine (kilograms)	Pseudoephedrine preparations[a] (kilograms)	Safrole (litres)
Africa																		
Côte d'Ivoire																		
2011	—	—	—	a	—	—	—	—	—	—	—	—	—	—	—	—	—	—
2012	—	—	—	a	—	—	—	—	—	—	—	—	—	—	—	—	—	—
2013	—	—	—	1	—	—	—	—	—	—	—	—	—	—	—	—	—	—
Kenya																		
2015	—	—	18	—	—	—	—	—	—	—	—	—	—	—	—	—	—	—
Mali																		
2015	—	—	12	—	—	—	—	—	—	—	—	—	—	—	—	—	—	—
Namibia																		
2014	—	—	21	—	—	—	2 100	—	—	—	—	—	—	—	—	—	—	—
Nigeria																		
2011	—	—	56	—	—	—	—	—	—	—	—	—	—	—	—	—	—	—
2012	—	—	461	—	—	—	—	—	—	—	—	—	—	—	—	—	—	—
United Republic of Tanzania																		
2014	—	—	4	—	—	—	—	—	—	—	—	—	—	—	—	—	—	—
Zambia																		
2014	—	—	—	—	—	—	—	—	—	—	—	—	—	—	—	—	—	—

PRECURSORS

Country	Year	Acetic anhydride (litres)	N-Acetylanthranilic acid (kilograms)	Ephedrine (kilograms)	Ephedrine preparations[a] (kilograms)	Ergometrine (grams)	Ergotamine (grams)	Isosafrole (litres)	Lysergic acid (grams)	3,4-Methylenedioxyphenyl-2-propanone (litres)	Norephedrine (phenylpropanolamine) (kilograms)	Phenylacetic acid (kilograms)	alpha-phenylacetoacetonitrile (APAAN)[b] (kilograms)	1-Phenyl-2-propanone (litres)	Piperonal (kilograms)	Potassium permanganate (kilograms)	Pseudoephedrine (kilograms)	Pseudoephedrine preparations[a] (kilograms)	Safrole (litres)
Zimbabwe	2013	–	–	–	–	–	–	–	–	–	–	–	–	–	–	–	–	–	–
	2014	–	–	70	113	–	–	–	–	–	–	–	–	–	–	–	–	–	–
Regional total	**2011**	0	0	56	0	0	0	0	0	0	0	0	0	0	0	0	0	0	0
	2012	0	0	461	0	0	0	0	0	0	0	0	0	0	0	0	0	0	0
	2013	0	0	0	114	0	0	0	0	0	0	0	0	0	0	0	0	0	0
	2014	0	0	95	0	0	0	2 100	0	0	0	0	0	0	0	0	0	0	0
	2015	0	0	31	0	0	0	0	0	0	0	0	0	0	0	0	0	0	0

Americas

Central America and the Caribbean

Country	Year	Acetic anhydride (litres)	N-Acetylanthranilic acid (kilograms)	Ephedrine (kilograms)	Ephedrine preparations[a] (kilograms)	Ergometrine (grams)	Ergotamine (grams)	Isosafrole (litres)	Lysergic acid (grams)	3,4-Methylenedioxyphenyl-2-propanone (litres)	Norephedrine (phenylpropanolamine) (kilograms)	Phenylacetic acid (kilograms)	alpha-phenylacetoacetonitrile (APAAN)[b] (kilograms)	1-Phenyl-2-propanone (litres)	Piperonal (kilograms)	Potassium permanganate (kilograms)	Pseudoephedrine (kilograms)	Pseudoephedrine preparations[a] (kilograms)	Safrole (litres)
Belize	2013	660	–	–	–	–	–	–	–	–	–	–	–	–	–	–	–	–	–
El Salvador	2011	512	–	–	–	–	–	–	–	–	–	–	–	–	–	–	–	–	–
Guatemala	2011	–	–	100	–	–	–	–	–	–	–	1	–	–	–	–	95	–	–
Honduras	2011	–	–	–	–	–	–	–	–	–	–	–	–	–	–	–	–	0	–
	2012	–	–	–	–	–	–	–	–	–	–	–	–	–	–	–	22 565	41	–
	2013	–	–	–	–	–	–	–	–	–	–	–	–	–	–	–	1	–	–
Nicaragua	2012	–	–	–	–	–	–	–	–	13	–	52	–	–	–	–	–	–	–

ANNEXES

Country / Year	Acetic anhydride (litres)	N-Acetylanthranilic acid (kilograms)	Ephedrine (kilograms)	Ephedrine preparations[a] (kilograms)	Ergometrine (grams)	Ergotamine (grams)	Isosafrole (litres)	Lysergic acid (grams)	3,4-Methylenedioxyphenyl-2-propanone (litres)	Norephedrine (phenylpropanolamine) (kilograms)	Phenylacetic acid (kilograms)	alpha-phenylacetoacetonitrile (APAAN)[b] (kilograms)	1-Phenyl-2-propanone (litres)	Piperonal (kilograms)	Potassium permanganate (kilograms)	Pseudoephedrine (kilograms)	Pseudoephedrine preparations[a] (kilograms)	Safrole (litres)
Panama																		
2013	—	—	—	—	—	—	—	—	—	22	—	—	—	—	—	—	—	—
Regional total																		
2011	512	0	100	0	0	0	0	0	0	0	1	0	0	0	0	95	42	0
2012	0	0	0	0	0	0	0	0	13	0	52	0	0	0	0	22 565	0	0
2013	660	0	0	0	0	0	0	0	0	22	0	0	0	0	0	1	0	0
2014	0	0	0	0	0	0	0	0	0	0	0	0	0	0	0	0	0	0
2015	0	0	0	0	0	0	0	0	0	0	0	0	0	0	0	0	0	0
North America																		
Canada																		
2011	—	—	13	—	—	—	—	7	—	—	—	—	—	—	1	11	—	65
2012	—	—	686	—	20	—	—	°	526	—	—	—	—	—	5	309	—	2 025
2013	4	—	—	—	—	—	—	—	—	—	—	—	—	—	—	—	—	—
2014	°	—	65	—	—	—	—	14	—	—	—	—	—	—	1	2	[b]	2
2015	°	—	°	[b]	—	—	—	°	°	—	—	—	—	—	—	°	—	°
Mexico																		
2011	76 625	—	2	—	—	—	—	—	2 184	—	14 370	—	—	°	—	313	—	2 371
2012	35 040	—	—	33 566	1 630	—	—	—	4 699	—	1 188	—	—	3	35	62	—	—
2013	7 597	—	—	—	—	—	—	—	2 796	—	3 324	—	—	—	—	7 197	—	—
2014	13 368	—	—	—	—	—	—	—	5 892	—	1 315	—	—	—	—	—	—	—
2015	3 356	—	—	—	820	—	—	3	16 537	—	550	—	—	—	—	—	—	—
United States of America																		
2011	24 713	—	17 520	—	—	—	—	3	200	°	997 330	—	—	—	224	2 502	[c]	2 281
2012	859	—	270	—	—	—	—	3	—	—	314	—	—	—	152	241	—	1

PRECURSORS

Country / Year	Acetic anhydride (litres)	N-Acetylanthranilic acid (kilograms)	Ephedrine (kilograms)	Ephedrine preparations[a] (kilograms)	Ergometrine (grams)	Ergotamine (grams)	Isosafrole (litres)	Lysergic acid (grams)	3,4-Methylenedioxyphenyl-2-propanone (litres)	Norephedrine (phenylpropanolamine) (kilograms)	Phenylacetic acid (kilograms)	alpha-phenylacetoacetonitrile (APAAN)[b] (kilograms)	1-Phenyl-2-propanone (litres)	Piperonal (kilograms)	Potassium permanganate (kilograms)	Pseudoephedrine (kilograms)	Pseudoephedrine preparations[a] (kilograms)	Safrole (litres)
2013	—	—	16	—	—	—	—	—	—	—	—	—	—	—	—	1 029	—	10
2014	°	—	1	°	—	—	—	—	—	—	—	—	—	—	—	19	1	—
2015	—	—	°	—	—	—	—	—	—	—	—	—	—	—	—	210	—	—
Regional total																		
2011	101 339	0	17 535	33 566	0	820	0	9	122	0	1 011 700	0	2 384	0	225	2 827	0	4 717
2012	35 900	0	956	0	0	1 650	0	3	0	0	1 502	0	5 225	3	192	612	0	2 026
2013	7 601	0	16	0	0	0	0	0	0	0	3 324	0	2 796	0	0	8 228	0	10
2014	13 368	0	65	0	0	0	0	14	0	0	1 315	0	5 893	0	1	19	1	2
2015	3 356	0	1	0	0	0	0	0	0	0	550	0	16 537	0	0	210	0	0
South America																		
Argentina																		
2011	—	—	—	—	—	—	—	—	—	—	—	—	—	—	12	250	—	—
2012	—	—	9	—	—	—	—	—	—	—	—	—	—	—	2	—	—	—
2013	—	—	—	1	—	—	—	—	—	—	—	—	—	—	2	—	—	—
2014	33	—	24	—	—	—	—	—	—	—	—	—	—	—	—	—	—	—
2015	1 044	—	47	—	—	—	—	—	—	—	—	—	—	—	56	—	—	—
Bolivia (Plurinational State of)																		
2011	—	—	°	—	—	—	—	—	—	—	—	—	—	—	9 914	°	—	—
2012	—	—	—	—	—	—	—	—	—	—	—	—	—	—	964	—	—	—
2013	—	—	—	—	—	—	—	—	—	—	—	—	—	—	3 058	—	—	—
2014	—	—	—	—	—	—	—	—	—	—	—	—	—	—	1 492	—	—	—
2015	—	—	—	—	—	—	—	—	—	—	—	—	—	—	862	—	—	—

Country	Year	Acetic anhydride (litres)	N-Acetylanthranilic acid (kilograms)	Ephedrine (kilograms)	Ephedrine preparations[a] (kilograms)	Ergometrine (grams)	Ergotamine (grams)	Isosafrole (litres)	Lysergic acid (grams)	3,4-Methylenedioxyphenyl-2-propanone (litres)	Norephedrine (phenylpropanolamine) (kilograms)	Phenylacetic acid (kilograms)	alpha-phenylacetoacetonitrile (APAAN)[b] (kilograms)	1-Phenyl-2-propanone (litres)	Piperonal (kilograms)	Potassium permanganate (kilograms)	Pseudoephedrine (kilograms)	Pseudoephedrine preparations[a] (kilograms)	Safrole (litres)
Brazil	2011	53	–	–	–	–	–	–	–	–	–	–	–	–	–	232	–	41	–
	2012	1 878	–	–	–	–	–	–	–	–	–	–	–	–	–	278	–	–	–
	2013	249	–	–	–	–	–	–	–	–	–	–	–	–	–	14 621	–	–	–
	2014	–	–	–	–	–	–	–	–	–	–	–	–	–	–	1	–	–	–
Chile	2015	–	–	–	0	–	–	–	–	–	–	–	–	–	–	–	–	–	–
Colombia	2011	–	–	–	–	–	–	–	–	–	–	–	–	–	–	24 044	–	–	–
	2012	11	–	–	–	–	–	–	–	–	–	–	–	–	–	55 677	–	–	–
	2013	–	–	–	–	–	–	–	–	–	–	–	–	–	–	21 873	–	–	–
	2014	–	–	–	–	–	–	–	–	–	–	–	–	–	–	166 291	–	–	–
	2015	8	–	–	–	–	–	–	–	–	–	–	–	–	–	57 639	–	–	–
Ecuador	2011	–	–	–	–	–	–	–	–	–	–	–	–	220	–	233	–	–	–
	2014	–	–	–	–	–	–	–	–	–	–	–	–	–	–	10	–	–	–
	2015	–	–	–	–	–	–	–	–	–	–	–	–	–	–	2	–	–	–
Paraguay	2013	–	–	–	–	–	–	–	–	–	–	–	–	–	–	3 705	–	–	–
Peru	2011	–	–	–	–	–	–	–	–	–	–	–	–	–	–	1 997	–	–	–
	2012	–	–	–	–	–	–	–	–	–	–	–	–	–	–	3 093	–	–	–

PRECURSORS

Country / Year	Acetic anhydride (litres)	N-Acetylanthranilic acid (kilograms)	Ephedrine (kilograms)	Ephedrine preparations[a] (kilograms)	Ergometrine (grams)	Ergotamine (grams)	Isosafrole (litres)	Lysergic acid (grams)	3,4-Methylenedioxyphenyl-2-propanone (litres)	Norephedrine (phenylpropanolamine) (kilograms)	Phenylacetic acid (kilograms)	alpha-phenylacetoacetonitrile (APAAN)[b] (kilograms)	1-Phenyl-2-propanone (litres)	Piperonal (kilograms)	Potassium permanganate (kilograms)	Pseudoephedrine (kilograms)	Pseudoephedrine preparations[a] (kilograms)	Safrole (litres)
2013	1	–	–	–	–	–	–	–	–	–	–	–	–	–	2 787	–	–	–
2014	15	–	–	–	–	–	–	–	–	–	–	–	–	–	2 735	–	–	–
2015	–	–	–	–	–	–	–	–	–	–	–	–	–	–	53	–	–	–
Venezuela (Bolivarian Republic of)																		
2011	–	–	–	16	–	–	–	–	–	–	–	–	–	–	100	–	3	–
2012	–	–	–	–	–	–	–	–	–	–	–	–	–	–	2 447	–	–	–
2014	–	–	–	–	–	–	–	–	–	–	–	–	–	–	1 120	–	–	–
2015	–	–	–	–	–	–	–	–	–	–	–	–	–	–	1 554	–	–	–
Regional total																		
2011	53	0	0	16	0	0	0	0	0	0	0	0	220	0	36 532	250	44	0
2012	1 890	0	9	0	0	0	0	0	0	0	0	0	0	0	62 462	0	0	0
2013	250	0	0	1	0	0	0	0	0	0	0	0	0	0	46 046	0	0	0
2014	48	0	24	0	0	0	0	0	0	0	0	0	0	0	171 649	0	0	0
2015	1 052	0	47	0	0	0	0	0	0	0	0	0	0	0	60 166	0	0	0

Asia

East and South-East Asia

Country / Year	Acetic anhydride (litres)	N-Acetylanthranilic acid (kilograms)	Ephedrine (kilograms)	Ephedrine preparations[a] (kilograms)	Ergometrine (grams)	Ergotamine (grams)	Isosafrole (litres)	Lysergic acid (grams)	3,4-Methylenedioxyphenyl-2-propanone (litres)	Norephedrine (phenylpropanolamine) (kilograms)	Phenylacetic acid (kilograms)	alpha-phenylacetoacetonitrile (APAAN)[b] (kilograms)	1-Phenyl-2-propanone (litres)	Piperonal (kilograms)	Potassium permanganate (kilograms)	Pseudoephedrine (kilograms)	Pseudoephedrine preparations[a] (kilograms)	Safrole (litres)
Cambodia																		
2011	–	–	3	–	–	–	–	–	–	–	–	–	–	–	–	6	–	2 058
China[d]																		
2011	16 946	–	4 210	–	–	–	–	–	–	–	4 520	–	–	–	–	–	–	–
2012	17 131	–	3 210	2 428	–	449	–	–	–	–	30	–	259	–	29 927	1 170	902	–
2013	94 948	–	11 103	5 718	–	–	–	–	18	–	6 552	–	5 434	–	3 521	908	–	–
2014	22 635	–	31 576	3 222	–	–	–	–	33	°	49 651	–	3 241	–	2 120	–	–	–
2015	11 070	°	23 480	221	–	–	–	–	°	6	3	–	5 407	–	31 550	13	–	–

Country / Year	Acetic anhydride (litres)	N-Acetylanthranilic acid (kilograms)	Ephedrine (kilograms)	Ephedrine preparations[a] (kilograms)	Ergometrine (grams)	Ergotamine (grams)	Isosafrole (litres)	Lysergic acid (grams)	3,4-Methylenedioxyphenyl-2-propanone (litres)	Norephedrine (phenylpropanolamine) (kilograms)	Phenylacetic acid (kilograms)	alpha-phenylacetoacetonitrile (APAAN)[b] (kilograms)	1-Phenyl-2-propanone (litres)	Piperonal (kilograms)	Potassium permanganate (kilograms)	Pseudoephedrine (kilograms)	Pseudoephedrine preparations[a] (kilograms)	Safrole (litres)
China, Hong Kong SAR																		
2012	—	—	—	—	—	—	—	—	—	—	—	—	—	—	—	33	—	—
2013	—	—	41	—	—	—	—	—	—	—	—	—	—	—	—	34	27[a]	—
China, Macao SAR																		
2012	—	—	—	167	—	—	—	—	—	—	—	—	—	—	—	—	—	—
2014	—	—	—	°	—	—	—	—	—	—	—	—	—	—	—	—	—	—
Indonesia																		
2011	—	—	—	[a]	—	—	—	—	—	—	—	—	—	—	—	—	40	—
2012	—	—	4	[a]	—	—	—	—	—	4	—	—	—	—	—	—	—	—
2013	—	—	°	—	—	—	—	—	—	—	—	—	—	—	—	—	—	257
2014	—	—	°	[a]	—	—	—	—	—	—	—	—	—	—	—	—	—	—
2015	—	—	—	°	—	—	—	—	—	—	—	—	—	—	—	—	[a]	—
Japan																		
2013	—	—	—	1	—	—	—	—	—	—	—	—	—	—	—	—	—	—
2014	—	—	5	—	—	—	—	—	—	—	—	—	—	—	—	6	—	—
2015	—	—	—	—	—	—	—	—	—	—	—	—	—	—	—	—	—	—
Lao People's Democratic Republic																		
2013	—	—	—	3	—	—	—	—	—	—	—	—	—	—	—	—	—	—
Malaysia																		
2011	—	—	109	—	—	—	—	—	—	—	—	—	—	—	—	903	—	7 675
2012	—	—	—	91	—	—	—	—	—	—	—	—	—	—	—	5	—	—
2013	—	—	66	90	—	—	—	—	—	—	—	—	—	—	—	—	63	—
2014	—	—	—	33	—	—	—	—	—	—	—	—	—	—	1	287	112	—
2015	—	—	75	—	—	—	—	—	—	—	—	—	—	—	—	56	—	—

PRECURSORS

Country	Year	Acetic anhydride (litres)	N-Acetylanthranilic acid (kilograms)	Ephedrine (kilograms)	Ephedrine preparations[a] (kilograms)	Ergometrine (grams)	Ergotamine (grams)	Isosafrole (litres)	Lysergic acid (grams)	3,4-Methylenedioxyphenyl-2-propanone (litres)	Norephedrine (phenylpropanolamine) (kilograms)	Phenylacetic acid (kilograms)	alpha-phenylacetoacetonitrile (APAAN)[b] (kilograms)	1-Phenyl-2-propanone (litres)	Piperonal (kilograms)	Potassium permanganate (kilograms)	Pseudoephedrine (kilograms)	Pseudoephedrine preparations[a] (kilograms)	Safrole (litres)
Myanmar	2013	–	–	–	133	–	–	–	–	–	–	95	–	4 800	–	–	–	3 581	–
	2014	–	–	–	–	–	–	–	–	–	–	–	–	–	–	–	–	–	–
	2015	60	–	°	–	–	–	–	–	–	–	–	–	–	–	–	–	–	–
Philippines	2011	–	–	106	–	–	–	–	–	–	–	–	–	–	–	–	°	–	–
	2012	–	–	378	–	–	–	–	–	212	273	–	–	–	1	–	3	–	–
	2013	–	–	1	–	–	–	–	–	–	°	–	–	–	°	–	609	–	–
	2014	–	–	510	–	–	–	–	–	–	°	–	–	–	–	–	–	–	–
	2015	–	–	50	–	–	–	–	–	–	–	–	–	–	–	–	2	–	–
Singapore	2011	–	–	–	–	–	–	–	–	–	–	–	–	–	–	–	–	155	–
Thailand	2011	–	–	3	–	–	–	–	–	–	–	–	–	–	–	–	–	1[a]	–
	2012	–	–	17	°	–	–	–	–	–	–	–	–	–	–	–	–	[a]	–
	2013	–	–	–	–	–	–	–	–	–	–	–	–	–	–	–	–	[a]	–
	2014	–	–	–	–	–	–	–	–	–	–	–	–	–	–	–	–	6	–
	2015	–	–	–	–	–	–	–	–	–	–	–	–	–	–	–	–	3	–
Viet Nam	2013	–	–	–	5	–	–	–	–	–	–	–	–	–	–	–	–	47	–
	2014	–	–	4	–	–	–	–	–	–	–	–	–	–	–	–	–	22	–
Regional total	2011	16 946	0	4 431	0	0	0	0	0	0	0	4 520	0	0	0	0	2 079	196	9 734
	2012	17 131	0	3 608	2 686	0	0	0	0	212	276	30	0	259	1	29 927	40	902	0

ANNEXES

Country / Year	Acetic anhydride (litres)	N-Acetylanthranilic acid (kilograms)	Ephedrine (kilograms)	Ephedrine preparations[a] (kilograms)	Ergometrine (grams)	Ergotamine (grams)	Isosafrole (litres)	Lysergic acid (grams)	3,4-Methylenedioxyphenyl-2-propanone (litres)	Norephedrine (phenylpropanolamine) (kilograms)	Phenylacetic acid (kilograms)	alpha-phenylacetoacetonitrile (APAAN)[b] (kilograms)	1-Phenyl-2-propanone (litres)	Piperonal (kilograms)	Potassium permanganate (kilograms)	Pseudoephedrine (kilograms)	Pseudoephedrine preparations[a] (kilograms)	Safrole (litres)
2013	94 948	0	11 211	5 950	0	449	0	0	18	0	6 647	0	5 434	0	3 521	1 551	3 718	257
2014	22 635	0	32 095	3 255	0	0	0	0	33	0	49 651	0	8 041	0	2 121	309	118	0
2015	11 130	0	23 604	221	0	0	0	0	0	6	3	0	5 407	0	31 550	77	3	0
South Asia																		
India																		
2011	–	–	6 308	104	–	–	–	62	–	–	–	–	–	–	–	118	676	–
2012	336	–	559	–	–	–	–	–	–	8	–	–	–	–	–	5 691	236	–
2013	242	–	707	–	–	–	–	–	–	–	–	–	78	–	–	5 098	–	–
2014	100	–	654	–	–	–	–	–	–	–	–	–	–	–	–	–	676	–
2015	4	–	97	[a]	–	–	–	472	43	–	–	–	–	–	–	730	[a]	–
Regional total																		
2011	0	0	6 308	104	0	0	0	62	0	0	0	0	0	0	0	118	676	0
2012	336	0	559	0	0	0	0	0	0	8	0	0	0	0	0	5 691	236	0
2013	242	0	707	0	0	0	0	0	0	0	0	0	78	0	0	5 098	0	0
2014	100	0	654	0	0	0	0	0	0	0	0	0	0	0	0	0	676	0
2015	4	0	97	0	0	0	0	472	43	0	0	0	0	0	0	730	0	0
West Asia																		
Afghanistan																		
2011	68 245	–	–	–	–	–	–	–	–	–	–	–	–	–	–	–	–	–
2012	31 451	–	–	–	–	–	–	–	–	–	–	–	–	–	–	–	–	–
2013	14 212	–	–	–	–	–	–	–	–	–	–	–	–	–	–	–	–	–
2014	7 751	–	–	–	–	–	–	–	–	–	–	–	–	–	–	–	–	–
2015	3 761	–	–	–	–	–	–	–	–	–	–	–	–	–	–	–	–	–

PRECURSORS

Country / Year	Acetic anhydride (litres)	N-Acetylanthranilic acid (kilograms)	Ephedrine (kilograms)	Ephedrine preparations[a] (kilograms)	Ergometrine (grams)	Ergotamine (grams)	Isosafrole (litres)	Lysergic acid (grams)	3,4-Methylenedioxyphenyl-2-propanone (litres)	Norephedrine (phenylpropanolamine) (kilograms)	Phenylacetic acid (kilograms)	alpha-phenylacetoacetonitrile (APAAN)[b] (kilograms)	1-Phenyl-2-propanone (litres)	Piperonal (kilograms)	Potassium permanganate (kilograms)	Pseudoephedrine (kilograms)	Pseudoephedrine preparations[a] (kilograms)	Safrole (litres)
Armenia																		
2011	1	–	–	–	–	–	–	–	–	–	–	–	–	–	–	–	–	–
2012	°	–	–	–	–	–	–	–	–	–	–	–	–	–	–	–	–	–
2013	°	–	–	–	–	–	–	–	–	–	–	–	–	–	–	–	–	–
2014	°	–	–	–	–	–	–	–	–	–	–	–	–	–	–	–	–	–
Iran (Islamic Republic of)[e]																		
2011	–	–	3 809	–	–	–	–	–	–	–	–	–	–	–	–	–	–	–
2013	16 501	–	–	–	–	–	–	–	–	–	–	–	–	–	–	–	–	–
Kazakhstan																		
2011	–	–	–	–	–	–	–	–	–	–	–	–	–	–	°	–	–	–
2015	–	–	–	–	–	–	–	–	–	–	–	–	–	–	13 401	–	–	–
Kyrgyzstan																		
2012	792	–	–	–	–	–	–	–	–	–	–	–	–	–	–	–	–	–
Lebanon																		
2012	–	–	6	20	–	–	–	–	–	–	–	–	–	–	–	–	–	–
2013	–	–	1	–	–	–	–	–	–	–	–	–	–	–	–	–	–	–
2014	–	–	–	[a]	–	–	–	–	–	–	–	–	–	–	–	–	[a]	–
2015	–	–	–	–	–	–	–	–	–	–	16 082	–	–	–	–	–	–	–
Pakistan																		
2011	43	–	295	–	–	–	–	–	–	–	–	–	–	–	1 250	–	–	–
2012	81	–	–	–	–	–	–	–	–	–	–	–	–	–	–	–	–	–
2013	15 480	–	53	–	–	–	–	–	–	–	–	–	–	–	–	–	–	–
2014	185	–	35	–	–	–	–	–	–	–	–	–	–	–	–	–	–	–
2015	5 319	–	–	–	–	–	–	–	–	–	–	–	–	–	–	–	–	–

ANNEXES

Country / Year	Acetic anhydride (litres)	N-Acetylanthranilic acid (kilograms)	Ephedrine (kilograms)	Ephedrine preparations[a] (kilograms)	Ergometrine (grams)	Ergotamine (grams)	Isosafrole (litres)	Lysergic acid (grams)	3,4-Methylenedioxyphenyl-2-propanone (litres)	Norephedrine (phenylpropanolamine) (kilograms)	Phenylacetic acid (kilograms)	alpha-phenylacetoacetonitrile (APAAN)[b] (kilograms)	1-Phenyl-2-propanone (litres)	Piperonal (kilograms)	Potassium permanganate (kilograms)	Pseudoephedrine (kilograms)	Pseudoephedrine preparations[a] (kilograms)	Safrole (litres)
Qatar																		
2013	–	–	–	–	–	–	–	–	–	–	–	–	–	–	1 600	–	–	–
Syrian Arab Republic																		
2012	–	–	–	–	–	–	–	–	–	–	–	–	498	–	–	–	–	–
Turkey																		
2011	3 706[f]	–	–	–	–	–	–	–	–	–	–	–	–	–	–	–	–	–
2012	177	–	–	0	–	–	–	–	–	–	–	–	–	–	–	–	–	–
2013	14 672	–	–	–	–	–	–	–	–	–	–	–	–	–	–	–	–	–
2014	854	–	33	–	–	–	–	–	–	–	–	–	–	–	–	–	–	–
2015	4 402	–	–	–	–	–	–	–	–	–	–	–	–	–	–	–	–	–
Uzbekistan																		
2011	–	–	–	–	–	–	–	–	–	–	–	–	–	–	3	–	–	–
2013	–	–	–	–	–	–	–	–	–	–	–	–	–	–	160	–	–	–
2014	–	–	–	–	–	–	–	–	–	–	–	–	–	–	52	–	–	–
2015	–	–	–	–	–	–	–	–	–	–	16 082	–	–	–	32 684	–	–	–
Regional total																		
2011	71 994	0	4 104	0	0	0	0	0	0	0	0	0	0	0	1 253	0	0	0
2012	32 501	0	6	20	0	0	0	0	0	0	0	0	498	0	0	0	0	0
2013	60 866	0	54	0	0	0	0	0	0	0	0	0	0	0	1 760	0	0	0
2014	8 790	0	68	0	0	0	0	0	0	0	0	0	0	0	52	0	0	0
2015	13 481	0	0	0	0	0	0	0	0	0	16 082	0	0	0	46 085	0	0	0

PRECURSORS

Europe
States not members of the European Union

Country / Year	Acetic anhydride (litres)	N-Acetylanthranilic acid (kilograms)	Ephedrine (kilograms)	Ephedrine preparations[a] (kilograms)	Ergometrine (grams)	Ergotamine (grams)	Isosafrole (litres)	Lysergic acid (grams)	3,4-Methylenedioxyphenyl-2-propanone (litres)	Norephedrine (phenylpropanolamine) (kilograms)	Phenylacetic acid (kilograms)	alpha-phenylacetoacetonitrile (APAAN)[b] (kilograms)	1-Phenyl-2-propanone (litres)	Piperonal (kilograms)	Potassium permanganate (kilograms)	Pseudoephedrine (kilograms)	Pseudoephedrine preparations[a] (kilograms)	Safrole (litres)
Belarus																		
2011	○	—	—	○	—	—	—	—	—	—	—	—	—	—	—	—	○	—
2012	—	—	—	—	—	—	—	—	—	—	—	—	—	—	—	—	○	—
2013	—	—	—	—	—	—	—	—	—	—	—	—	—	—	—	—	○	—
2014	—	—	—	—	—	—	—	—	—	—	—	—	—	—	—	1	—	—
2015	—	—	—	—	—	—	—	—	—	—	—	—	—	—	—	—	○	—
Norway																		
2012	—	—	—	1	—	—	—	—	—	—	—	—	—	—	—	—	—	—
2013	—	—	—	—	—	—	—	—	—	—	—	—	—	—	1	—	—	2
2014	—	—	—	—	—	—	—	—	—	—	—	—	○	—	—	—	—	—
2015	—	—	—	○	—	—	—	—	—	—	—	—	—	—	—	—	○	—
Republic of Moldova																		
2013	—	—	○	○	—	—	—	—	—	—	—	—	—	—	—	—	—	—
2014	—	—	○	—	—	—	—	—	—	—	—	—	—	—	—	—	[a]	—
2015	—	—	2	—	—	—	—	—	—	—	—	—	—	—	—	—	[a]	—
Russian Federation																		
2011	820	—	○	—	—	—	—	—	—	—	—	—	1 060	—	—	—	—	—
2012	5	—	○	○	—	—	—	—	—	—	—	—	4	—	—	3	—	—
2013	8	—	2	—	—	—	—	83	—	—	—	—	30	—	—	—	—	—
2014	17	—	—	○	—	—	—	—	—	—	—	—	○	—	—	—	○	—
2015	47	—	○	—	—	—	—	—	—	—	—	—	—	—	—	—	○	—

78

ANNEXES

Country	Year	Acetic anhydride (litres)	N-Acetylanthranilic acid (kilograms)	Ephedrine (kilograms)	Ephedrine preparations[a] (kilograms)	Ergometrine (grams)	Ergotamine (grams)	Isosafrole (litres)	Lysergic acid (grams)	3,4-Methylenedioxyphenyl-2-propanone (litres)	Norephedrine (phenylpropanolamine) (kilograms)	Phenylacetic acid (kilograms)	alpha-phenylacetoacetonitrile (APAAN)[b] (kilograms)	1-Phenyl-2-propanone (litres)	Piperonal (kilograms)	Potassium permanganate (kilograms)	Pseudoephedrine (kilograms)	Pseudoephedrine preparations[a] (kilograms)	Safrole (litres)
Serbia	2012	–	–	0	–	–	–	–	–	–	–	–	–	–	0	–	–	–	–
Switzerland	2014	–	–	–	–	a	–	–	–	–	–	–	–	–	–	–	–	–	–
Ukraine	2011	31	–	4	5	–	–	–	–	–	0	–	–	5	–	396	2	2	–
	2012	52	–	–	0	–	–	–	–	–	0	–	–	0	–	101	0	–	–
	2013	1 664	–	–	51	–	–	–	–	–	0	–	–	–	–	225	–	2 991	–
	2015	57	–	–	1	–	–	–	–	–	0	25	–	–	0	10	0	47	0

States members of the European Union

Country	Year	Acetic anhydride (litres)	N-Acetylanthranilic acid (kilograms)	Ephedrine (kilograms)	Ephedrine preparations[a] (kilograms)	Ergometrine (grams)	Ergotamine (grams)	Isosafrole (litres)	Lysergic acid (grams)	3,4-Methylenedioxyphenyl-2-propanone (litres)	Norephedrine (phenylpropanolamine) (kilograms)	Phenylacetic acid (kilograms)	alpha-phenylacetoacetonitrile (APAAN)[b] (kilograms)	1-Phenyl-2-propanone (litres)	Piperonal (kilograms)	Potassium permanganate (kilograms)	Pseudoephedrine (kilograms)	Pseudoephedrine preparations[a] (kilograms)	Safrole (litres)
Austria	2013	2	–	–	–	–	–	–	–	–	–	–	–	–	–	–	–	–	–
	2014	–	–	–	–	–	–	–	–	104	–	–	–	–	–	–	–	–	–
	2015	2 037	–	–	–	–	–	–	–	–	–	–	–	–	–	–	–	–	–
Belgium	2011	–	–	–	–	–	–	–	–	–	–	–	–	–	–	1	–	–	1
	2012	–	–	1	–	–	–	–	–	2 781	–	–	–	503	–	1	–	–	–
	2013	–	–	2	–	–	–	–	–	5	–	–	–	15	–	–	–	–	–
	2014	–	–	–	–	–	–	–	–	–	–	–	122	25	–	–	–	–	–
	2015	–	–	–	–	–	–	–	–	–	–	–	637	435	–	–	–	–	1
Bulgaria	2011	20	–	–	–	–	–	–	–	–	–	–	–	545	–	–	–	–	–
	2012	42	–	0	a	–	–	–	–	–	–	97	–	2	–	–	–	a	–
	2013	–	–	–	–	–	–	–	–	–	–	–	–	–	–	–	–	108	–

PRECURSORS

Country	Year	Acetic anhydride (litres)	N-Acetylanthranilic acid (kilograms)	Ephedrine (kilograms)	Ephedrine preparations[a] (kilograms)	Ergometrine (grams)	Ergotamine (grams)	Isosafrole (litres)	Lysergic acid (grams)	3,4-Methylenedioxyphenyl-2-propanone (litres)	Norephedrine (phenylpropanolamine) (kilograms)	Phenylacetic acid (kilograms)	alpha-phenylacetoacetonitrile (APAAN)[b] (kilograms)	1-Phenyl-2-propanone (litres)	Piperonal (kilograms)	Potassium permanganate (kilograms)	Pseudoephedrine (kilograms)	Pseudoephedrine preparations[a] (kilograms)	Safrole (litres)
	2014	—	—	—	—	—	—	—	—	—	—	—	1 980	—	—	—	—	841	—
	2015	—	—	32	—	—	—	—	—	—	—	—	—	—	—	—	—	66	—
Croatia	2011	—	—	°	°	—	—	—	—	—	—	—	—	—	—	—	—	—	—
	2013	—	—	—	°	—	—	—	—	—	—	—	—	—	—	—	—	—	—
	2014	—	—	—	°	—	—	—	—	—	—	—	—	°	—	—	—	°	—
Czechia[g]	2011	—	—	4	[a]	—	—	—	—	—	—	—	—	—	—	—	6	[a]	—
	2012	—	—	3	—	—	—	—	—	—	—	—	—	—	—	—	2	16	—
	2013	—	—	°	—	—	—	—	—	—	—	—	—	—	—	—	64	25	—
	2014	—	—	14	2	—	—	—	—	—	—	—	—	—	—	—	12	351	—
	2015	—	—	—	—	—	—	—	—	—	—	—	—	—	—	—	—	77	—
Estonia	2011	—	—	—	—	—	—	—	—	—	—	—	—	10	—	—	—	—	—
	2013	°	—	—	°	—	—	—	—	—	—	100	5	°	—	—	—	—	—
	2014	°	—	—	—	—	—	—	—	—	—	—	—	—	—	—	—	—	—
	2015	—	—	—	—	—	—	—	—	—	—	—	—	°	—	—	—	—	—
Finland	2011	—	—	—	[a]	—	—	—	—	—	—	—	—	3	—	—	—	—	—
	2012	—	—	—	[a]	—	—	—	—	—	—	—	—	°	—	—	—	°	—
	2013	—	—	—	600	—	—	—	—	—	—	—	—	—	°	—	—	—	—
	2014	—	—	—	°	—	—	—	—	—	—	—	—	—	—	—	—	—	—
	2015	—	—	—	2	—	—	—	—	—	—	—	—	°	—	—	—	°	—

ANNEXES

Country	Year	Acetic anhydride (litres)	N-Acetylanthranilic acid (kilograms)	Ephedrine (kilograms)	Ephedrine preparations[a] (kilograms)	Ergometrine (grams)	Ergotamine (grams)	Isosafrole (litres)	Lysergic acid (grams)	3,4-Methylenedioxyphenyl-2-propanone (litres)	Norephedrine (phenylpropanolamine) (kilograms)	Phenylacetic acid (kilograms)	alpha-phenylacetoacetonitrile (APAAN)[b] (kilograms)	1-Phenyl-2-propanone (litres)	Piperonal (kilograms)	Potassium permanganate (kilograms)	Pseudoephedrine (kilograms)	Pseudoephedrine preparations[a] (kilograms)	Safrole (litres)
France	2011	—	—	1	—	—	—	—	—	—	—	—	—	—	—	—	—	—	—
	2012	—	—	1	—	—	—	—	—	—	—	—	—	—	—	1	1	—	—
	2013	—	—	°	—	—	—	—	—	—	—	—	—	—	—	—	°	—	—
	2014	—	—	15	—	—	—	—	—	—	—	—	—	1	—	—	—	—	—
	2015	—	—	1	—	—	—	—	—	—	—	—	—	—	—	—	—	—	—
Germany	2011	3	—	20	—	—	—	—	—	—	—	6 000	—	24	—	—	3	[a]	—
	2012	—	—	°	—	—	—	—	—	—	—	—	—	38	—	°	—	—	—
	2013	—	—	1	[a]	—	—	—	—	—	—	—	5 105	°	—	1	—	[a]	—
	2014	—	—	°	°	—	—	—	—	—	—	—	38	2	—	1	—	—	—
	2015	1	—	4	—	—	—	—	—	—	—	—	—	2	°	°	°	[a]	—
Greece	2011	—	—	—	[a]	—	—	—	—	—	—	—	—	—	—	—	—	—	—
	2012	—	—	°	—	—	—	—	—	—	—	—	—	—	—	—	—	—	—
	2013	—	—	°	—	—	—	—	—	—	—	—	—	—	—	—	—	—	—
Hungary	2011	1	—	—	1	—	—	—	—	—	—	—	—	—	—	°	—	—	—
	2012	33	—	—	°	—	—	—	—	—	—	—	—	—	4	—	—	—	—
	2013	—	—	°	—	—	—	—	—	—	—	—	—	—	—	—	—	—	—
	2014	—	—	—	1	—	—	—	—	—	—	—	—	—	—	—	—	—	—
	2015	—	—	—	°	—	—	—	—	—	—	—	—	14	—	—	—	—	—

PRECURSORS

Country	Year	Acetic anhydride (litres)	N-Acetylanthranilic acid (kilograms)	Ephedrine (kilograms)	Ephedrine preparations[a] (kilograms)	Ergometrine (grams)	Ergotamine (grams)	Isosafrole (litres)	Lysergic acid (grams)	3,4-Methylenedioxyphenyl-2-propanone (litres)	Norephedrine (phenylpropanolamine) (kilograms)	Phenylacetic acid (kilograms)	alpha-phenylacetoacetonitrile (APAAN)[b] (kilograms)	1-Phenyl-2-propanone (litres)	Piperonal (kilograms)	Potassium permanganate (kilograms)	Pseudoephedrine (kilograms)	Pseudoephedrine preparations[a] (kilograms)	Safrole (litres)
Ireland	2011	—	—	—	3	—	—	—	449	—	—	—	—	—	—	—	—	—	—
	2012	—	—	—	—	—	—	—	—	3	—	—	—	—	—	—	—	—	—
	2014	—	—	°	—	—	—	—	—	—	—	—	—	22	—	—	—	—	—
	2015	—	—	—	—	—	—	—	—	—	—	—	—	—	—	—	—	—	—
Latvia	2011	°	—	—	°	—	—	—	—	—	—	—	—	—	—	—	—	—	—
Lithuania	2011	—	—	—	—	—	—	—	—	1	—	—	—	600	°	—	—	—	—
	2012	—	—	—	—	—	—	—	—	—	—	—	—	17	332	—	—	—	—
	2013	—	—	—	—	—	—	—	—	—	—	—	—	15	—	—	—	—	13
	2014	—	—	—	—	—	—	—	—	—	—	—	—	690	—	—	—	—	—
	2015	—	—	—	—	—	—	—	—	—	—	—	—	—	—	—	—	—	—
Luxembourg	2012	—	—	—	—	—	—	—	—	—	—	—	—	—	—	—	300	—	—
Netherlands	2011	—	—	—	—	—	—	—	—	—	—	—	—	111	—	—	—	—	105
	2012	—	—	—	—	—	—	10	—	112	—	—	—	123	—	—	500	—	—
	2013	—	—	—	—	—	—	10	—	507	—	—	—	—	—	—	—	—	—
	2014	—	—	—	—	—	—	—	—	—	—	—	3 090	428	5	80	—	—	13 825
	2015	—	—	—	—	—	—	—	—	—	—	258	710	525	45	26	—	2	2
Poland	2011	1	—	—	—	—	—	—	—	—	—	—	—	350	—	—	290	—	—
	2012	1 755	—	—	—	—	—	—	—	—	—	116	—	149	—	—	—	—	—

ANNEXES

Country	Year	Acetic anhydride (litres)	N-Acetylanthranilic acid (kilograms)	Ephedrine (kilograms)	Ephedrine preparations[a] (kilograms)	Ergometrine (grams)	Ergotamine (grams)	Isosafrole (litres)	Lysergic acid (grams)	3,4-Methylenedioxyphenyl-2-propanone (litres)	Norephedrine (phenylpropanolamine) (kilograms)	Phenylacetic acid (kilograms)	alpha-phenylacetoacetonitrile (APAAN)[b] (kilograms)	1-Phenyl-2-propanone (litres)	Piperonal (kilograms)	Potassium permanganate (kilograms)	Pseudoephedrine (kilograms)	Pseudoephedrine preparations[a] (kilograms)	Safrole (litres)
	2013	°	1	10	—	—	—	—	—	—	—	—	—	—	—	5	a	—	—
	2014	4	—	°	—	—	—	—	—	—	—	—	611	1 472	—	—	1	—	—
	2015	—	—	1	—	—	—	—	—	—	—	—	31	6 920	—	—	—	35	—
Portugal																			
	2013	—	—	1	—	—	—	—	—	—	—	—	—	—	—	—	°	—	—
	2015	—	—	°	—	—	—	—	—	—	—	—	—	—	—	—	—	—	—
Romania																			
	2013	—	—	—	—	—	—	—	—	—	—	—	—	—	1	—	—	—	—
	2014	—	—	—	—	—	—	—	—	—	—	—	150	—	—	—	—	—	—
Slovakia																			
	2011	6 020	—	—	—	—	—	—	—	—	—	—	—	—	—	—	a	—	—
	2012	—	—	°	—	—	—	—	—	—	—	—	—	—	—	—	°	—	—
	2013	—	—	°	—	—	—	—	—	—	—	—	—	—	—	—	°	—	—
	2014	—	—	°	—	—	—	—	—	—	—	—	—	—	—	°	—	a	—
	2015	—	—	°	—	—	—	—	—	—	—	—	—	—	—	1 000	°	11	—
Slovenia																			
	2012	—	—	°	°	—	—	—	—	°	—	—	—	—	—	°	—	—	—
	2013	—	—	°	—	—	—	—	—	—	—	—	—	—	—	—	—	—	—
Spain																			
	2011	—	—	1 500	—	—	—	—	—	—	—	—	—	—	—	1	—	—	—
	2012	11	—	—	—	—	1	—	—	—	—	—	—	—	1 400	19	—	—	—
	2013	9 497	—	—	—	—	—	—	—	—	—	—	—	—	—	5 926	—	—	—
	2014	110	—	—	—	—	—	—	—	—	—	—	—	—	—	—	—	—	—
	2015	1	—	2	—	—	—	—	—	—	—	2	122	—	—	—	—	—	—

PRECURSORS

Country / Year	Acetic anhydride (litres)	N-Acetylanthranilic acid (kilograms)	Ephedrine (kilograms)	Ephedrine preparations[a] (kilograms)	Ergometrine (grams)	Ergotamine (grams)	Isosafrole (litres)	Lysergic acid (grams)	3,4-Methylenedioxyphenyl-2-propanone (litres)	Norephedrine (phenylpropanolamine) (kilograms)	Phenylacetic acid (kilograms)	alpha-phenylacetoacetonitrile (APAAN)[b] (kilograms)	1-Phenyl-2-propanone (litres)	Piperonal (kilograms)	Potassium permanganate (kilograms)	Pseudoephedrine (kilograms)	Pseudoephedrine preparations[a] (kilograms)	Safrole (litres)
Sweden																		
2011	6 894	–	–	2	–	–	–	–	–	–	–	–	–	–	–	–	–	–
2012	1 899	–	0	1	–	–	–	–	–	–	–	–	–	0	–	–	–	–
2013	11 171	–	–	1[a]	–	–	–	–	–	–	–	–	–	–	–	–	–	–
2014	131	–	–	3	–	–	–	–	–	–	–	–	–	–	–	–	–	–
2015	2 144	–	–	1	–	–	–	–	–	–	–	–	–	–	–	–	–	–
United Kingdom																		
2011	–	–	500	[a]	–	–	–	–	–	–	–	–	–	10	–	–	–	–
2012	–	1	–	–	–	–	–	–	–	–	–	–	–	–	–	–	–	–
2013	–	–	–	–	–	–	–	–	–	–	–	–	–	–	–	–	–	–
Regional total																		
2011	6 894	0	530	11	0	0	0	449	1	1	6 000	0	2 708	10	396	304	2	106
2012	1 899	1	1 504	2	0	0	10	0	3	0	116	0	836	332	121	804	16	0
2013	11 171	1	15	653	0	1	10	83	3 910	0	97	0	61	1 405	6 240	64	–	13 848
2014	131	0	31	7	0	0	0	0	5	0	100	11 062	2 640	5	1	13	3 125	0
2015	2 144	0	7	3	0	0	0	0	507	0	286	1 537	7 896	45	1 036	32	225	3

Oceania

Country / Year	Acetic anhydride (litres)	N-Acetylanthranilic acid (kilograms)	Ephedrine (kilograms)	Ephedrine preparations[a] (kilograms)	Ergometrine (grams)	Ergotamine (grams)	Isosafrole (litres)	Lysergic acid (grams)	3,4-Methylenedioxyphenyl-2-propanone (litres)	Norephedrine (phenylpropanolamine) (kilograms)	Phenylacetic acid (kilograms)	alpha-phenylacetoacetonitrile (APAAN)[b] (kilograms)	1-Phenyl-2-propanone (litres)	Piperonal (kilograms)	Potassium permanganate (kilograms)	Pseudoephedrine (kilograms)	Pseudoephedrine preparations[a] (kilograms)	Safrole (litres)
Australia																		
2011	6	–	261	5	4	–	°	–	1	1	10	–	–	°	–	724	723	2 565
2012	2	–	520	–	–	207	°	691	°	2	°	–	1	°	–	770	2	1
2013	–	–	1 253	–	–	57	–	523	–	1	°	–	1	°	–	629	–	11
2014	–	–	457	–	–	281	°	–	20	°	1	–	–	1	–	11	–	184
2015	–	–	457	–	–	–	–	–	139	12	–	–	–	–	–	72	–	73

ANNEXES

Country / Year	Acetic anhydride (litres)	N-Acetylanthranilic acid (kilograms)	Ephedrine (kilograms)	Ephedrine preparations[a] (kilograms)	Ergometrine (grams)	Ergotamine (grams)	Isosafrole (litres)	Lysergic acid (grams)	3,4-Methylenedioxyphenyl-2-propanone (litres)	Norephedrine (phenylpropanolamine) (kilograms)	Phenylacetic acid (kilograms)	alpha-phenylacetoacetonitrile (APAAN)[b] (kilograms)	1-Phenyl-2-propanone (litres)	Piperonal (kilograms)	Potassium permanganate (kilograms)	Pseudoephedrine (kilograms)	Pseudoephedrine preparations[a] (kilograms)	Safrole (litres)
New Zealand																		
2011	○	—	—	96[a]	—	—	—	—	—	—	—	—	—	—	○	—	608[a]	—
2012	○	—	—	5	—	—	—	—	—	—	—	—	—	—	○	—	426[a]	1
2013	○	—	—	3[a]	—	—	—	—	—	—	—	—	—	—	○	—	691[a]	—
2015	3	—	952	—	—	—	—	—	—	—	—	—	—	—	—	61	—	—
Regional total																		
2011	6	0	261	101	0	4	0	0	1	1	10	0	0	0	0	724	1 332	2 565
2012	2	0	520	5	0	0	0	691	0	2	0	0	0	0	0	770	429	2
2013	0	0	1 253	3	0	207	0	523	0	1	0	0	1	0	0	629	691	11
2014	0	0	457	0	0	57	0	0	20	0	0	0	1	0	0	11	0	184
2015	3	0	1 409	0	0	281	0	0	139	1	1	0	0	1	0	133	0	73
World total																		
2011	197 744	0	33 326	33 797	0	824	0	521	124	2	1 022 231	0	5 312	10	38 406	6 398	2 291	17 122
2012	89 657	1	7 624	2 714	0	1 650	10	694	228	286	1 700	0	6 818	336	92 702	30 481	1 583	2 028
2013	175 739	1	13 256	6 721	0	657	10	606	3 927	23	10 068	0	8 292	1 405	57 567	15 571	7 534	14 117
2014	45 071	0	33 491	3 261	0	57	2 100	14	58	0	51 066	11 062	16 653	5	173 824	351	2 002	185
2015	31 169	0	25 196	224	0	281	0	472	689	18	16 922	1 537	29 840	46	138 837	1 182	228	77

[a] Seizures of ephedrine and pseudoephedrine reported to the Board in consumption units (such as tablets and doses) have not been converted into kilograms, as the actual quantity of ephedrine and pseudoephedrine is not known. The following countries have reported seizures of preparations containing ephedrine and/or pseudoephedrine quantified in terms of consumption units:

	Year	Ephedrine preparations (units)	Pseudoephedrine preparations (units)
Bulgaria	2012	50 000	3 660
Canada	2015	30 433	907
China, Hong Kong SAR	2013	—	656 271
Chile	2011	23 962	—
Côte d'Ivoire	2012	80 820	—

PRECURSORS

	Year	Ephedrine preparations (units)	Pseudoephedrine preparations (units)
Czechia[g]	2011	2 570	872 703
Finland	2011	6 107	–
	2012	6 359	–
Germany	2011	–	1 890
	2013	4 034	78
	2015	–	1 779
Greece	2011	8	–
India	2015	560	3 342 792
Indonesia	2011	3 000	–
	2012	53	–
	2014	17	–
	2015	–	60
Lebanon	2014	47	7 662
New Zealand	2011	123 431	34 833
	2012	–	3 630
	2013	6 956	5 073
Republic of Moldova	2014	–	60
	2015	–	60
Slovakia	2011	–	1 734
	2013	–	16 128
Sweden	2012	60 976	–
Switzerland	2014	185	–
Thailand	2011	–	10 240 820
	2012	–	2 011 100
	2013	–	302 630
United Kingdom	2011	288 000	–
	2013	–	1 000
United States	2011	–	4 003 371

[b] Included in Table I of the 1988 Convention, effective 6 October 2014.
[c] Figures reported for the United States for 2011 may inadvertently include sizeable seizures of *Sida cordifolia* and/or *Ephedra* plant extracts and are thus not comparable with figures for previous years.
[d] For statistical purposes, the data for China do not include those for China, Hong Kong Special Administrative Region (SAR), and China, Macao SAR.
[e] Based on data on seizures of precursors reported annually since 2010 by the Drug Control Headquarters of the Islamic Republic of Iran in the *Drug Control Report*.
[f] Turkish National Police, Anti-Smuggling and Organized Crime Department, *Turkish Report of Anti-Smuggling and Organized Crime: 2011* (Ankara, 2012).
[g] Since 17 May 2016, "Czechia" has replaced "Czech Republic" as the short name used in the United Nations.

Table A.2. Seizures of substances in Table II of the 1988 Convention as reported to the International Narcotics Control Board, 2011-2015

Country or territory, by region	Year	Acetone (litres)	Anthranilic acid (kilograms)	Ethyl ether (litres)	Hydrochloric acid (litres)	Methyl ethyl ketone (litres)	Piperidine (litres)	Sulphuric acid (litres)	Toluene (litres)
Africa									
Nigeria	2011	400	—	—	—	—	—	25	200
Regional total	2011	400	0	0	0	0	0	25	200
	2012	0	0	0	0	0	0	0	0
	2013	0	0	0	0	0	0	0	0
	2014	0	0	0	0	0	0	0	0
	2015	0	0	0	0	0	0	0	0
Americas									
Central America and the Caribbean									
Guatemala	2011	—	—	—	8 707	—	—	212	—
Honduras	2011	—	—	—	a	—	—	—	—
Regional total	2011	0	0	0	8 707	0	0	212	0
	2012	0	0	0	0	0	0	0	0
	2013	0	0	0	0	0	0	0	0
	2014	0	0	0	0	0	0	0	0
	2015	0	0	0	0	0	0	0	0
North America									
Canada	2011	371	—	49	274	4	°	201	1 825
	2012	2 786	—	°	855	4	18	24	1 718

PRECURSORS

Country or territory, by region	Year	Acetone (litres)	Anthranilic acid (kilograms)	Ethyl ether (litres)	Hydrochloric acid (litres)	Methyl ethyl ketone (litres)	Piperidine (litres)	Sulphuric acid (litres)	Toluene (litres)
	2013	569	–	–	48	–	–	2	981
	2014	940	–	–	219	–	–	153	645
	2015	°	°	–	°	°	°	°	–
Mexico									
	2011	23 262	–	219	78 125	–	–	1 652	49 410
	2012	10 669	–	14	29 310	64	–	3 171	26 243
	2013	6 901	–	28 001	14 207	94	–	439	12 333
	2014	2 402	–	°	8 446	281	–	1 406	4 324
	2015	8 117	–	–	188 256	184	–	4 508	26 643
United States of America									
	2011	71 142	–	115	109 602	29	11	1 231 111	262
	2012	10 594	–	60	206	3	189	125	12
	2013	2 457	–	18	1 681	11	57	1 930	102
	2014	4 477	–	277	1 326	11	57	1	72
	2015	3 810	–	168	1 325	18	–	1 244	41
Regional total									
	2011	**94 775**	**0**	**384**	**188 001**	**32**	**12**	**1 232 965**	**51 497**
	2012	**24 049**	**0**	**74**	**30 372**	**71**	**207**	**3 320**	**27 972**
	2013	**9 926**	**0**	**28 019**	**15 936**	**104**	**57**	**2 371**	**13 415**
	2014	**7 819**	**0**	**278**	**9 991**	**292**	**57**	**1 560**	**5 041**
	2015	**11 927**	**0**	**168**	**189 581**	**202**	**0**	**5 752**	**26 684**
South America									
Argentina									
	2011	245	–	182	96	2	–	16	–
	2012	311	–	131	52	53	–	26	–
	2013	2 768	–	104	165	3	–	202	–

ANNEXES

Country or territory, by region	Year	Acetone (litres)	Anthranilic acid (kilograms)	Ethyl ether (litres)	Hydrochloric acid (litres)	Methyl ethyl ketone (litres)	Piperidine (litres)	Sulphuric acid (litres)	Toluene (litres)
	2014	67	–	77	24 677	–	–	50	–
	2015	8 001	–	72	54 250	12	–	4 145	71 478
Bolivia (Plurinational State of)									
	2011	51 663	–	87	9 307	176	–	201 621	5 590
	2012	59 711	–	7 120	5 873	680	–	72 034	6 349
	2013	99 315	–	–	24 839	57	–	67 929	140
	2014	18 830	–	1 112	5 700	–	–	56 283	126
	2015	45 869	–	12 309	5 722	–	–	51 837	160
Brazil									
	2011	954	–	128	7 211	96	–	4 747	49
	2012	1 606	–	466	91 697	3 308	–	28 271	3 742
	2013	2 491	–	58	5 948	–	–	698	–
	2014	154	–	–	15 319	–	–	399	–
	2015	1 081	–	313	374 679	–	–	317 998	–
Chile									
	2011	–	–	–	19	–	–	93	–
	2012	–	–	–	–	–	–	5	–
	2013	2	–	–	144	–	–	63 610	–
	2014	25	–	4	226	–	–	233	–
	2015	°	–	–	142	14	–	196	°
Colombia									
	2011	463 883	–	1 541	96 660	–	–	201 812	42 044
	2012	739 247	–	25 295	76 290	1 419	–	163 242	33 792
	2013	482 063	–	2 286	144 686	3 406	–	1 060 578	765
	2014	456 643	–	2 117	75 058	6 155	–	276 004	191 390
	2015	613 920	–	11 697	211 090	172	–	282 853	56 221

PRECURSORS

Country or territory, by region	Year	Acetone (litres)	Anthranilic acid (kilograms)	Ethyl ether (litres)	Hydrochloric acid (litres)	Methyl ethyl ketone (litres)	Piperidine (litres)	Sulphuric acid (litres)	Toluene (litres)
Ecuador	2011	–	–	–	931	2 400	–	3 954	–
	2012	–	–	–	–	–	–	771	–
	2013	–	–	–	104	1 420	–	1 625	–
	2014	–	–	–	154	–	–	708	–
	2015	–	–	–	11	–	–	2 642	–
Paraguay	2011	4 500	–	5	833	–	–	5 229	2 650
	2013	–	–	–	2 019	–	–	6 960	–
Peru	2011	32 456	–	45	145 850	310	–	28 505	1 919
	2012	70 024	–	–	87 695	–	–	29 777	100
	2013	86 313	–	128	73 200	157	–	87 675	–
	2014	83 006	–	4	58 907	1 225	–	87 305	3 128
	2015	55 229	–	–	9 904	–	–	16 576	–
Venezuela (Bolivarian Republic of)	2011	15 858	–	–	25 781	1 140	–	30 284	1 200
	2012	39 331	–	–	28 605	–	–	87 470	427
	2013	27 598	–	–	1 061	99	–	831	301
	2015	203 824	–	–	19 318	–	–	10 411	10 666
Regional total	**2011**	**569 558**	**0**	**1 987**	**286 687**	**4 123**	**0**	**476 261**	**53 452**
	2012	**910 230**	**0**	**33 012**	**290 212**	**5 460**	**0**	**381 596**	**44 411**
	2013	**672 952**	**0**	**2 577**	**251 104**	**5 043**	**0**	**1 289 277**	**905**
	2014	**586 323**	**0**	**3 313**	**181 101**	**7 479**	**0**	**421 813**	**194 946**
	2015	**927 924**	**0**	**24 391**	**675 116**	**198**	**0**	**686 659**	**138 525**

ANNEXES

Country or territory, by region	Year	Acetone (litres)	Anthranilic acid (kilograms)	Ethyl ether (litres)	Hydrochloric acid (litres)	Methyl ethyl ketone (litres)	Piperidine (litres)	Sulphuric acid (litres)	Toluene (litres)
Asia									
East and South-East Asia									
China[b]	2011	21 474	–	17 980	150 165	1 391	–	23 024	–
	2012	31 953	–	15 770	166 825	1 217	–	18 479	13 900
	2013	351 870	490 302	12 204	1 627 816	1 906	2	1 297 043	221 026
	2014	139 171	816	7 918	1 659 718	640	–	679 966	290 917
	2015	9 768	9 575	909	565 575	727	–	177 115	91 804
Indonesia	2011	2	–	–	10	–	–	1	3
	2012	2	–	–	6	–	–	5	–
	2013	1	–	–	–	–	–	–	–
	2014	1	–	–	2 376	–	–	1 015	506
	2015	20	–	–	29	–	–	63	19
Malaysia	2011	800	–	45	800	–	–	–	950
	2012	460	–	–	300	–	–	100	150
	2013	85	–	9	219	–	–	–	25
	2014	139	–	13	779	–	–	–	153
	2015	194	–	3	283	–	–	–	513
Myanmar	2013	–	–	600	145	–	–	924	–
	2014	193 922	–	–	1 687 325	–	–	6 716 899	2 452 409
Philippines	2011	21	–	°	11	–	–	1	31 313
	2012	6 436	–	5	1 646	25	–	3 080	17 941
	2013	–	–	–	–	–	–	10	–

Country or territory, by region	Year	Acetone (litres)	Anthranilic acid (kilograms)	Ethyl ether (litres)	Hydrochloric acid (litres)	Methyl ethyl ketone (litres)	Piperidine (litres)	Sulphuric acid (litres)	Toluene (litres)
Singapore	2014	°	–	–	°	–	–	–	640
	2015	217	–	–	283	–	–	5	1 293
Singapore	2014	20	–	–	–	–	–	–	–
Thailand	2011	1	–	–	°	–	–	163	1
	2012	300	–	–	–	–	–	–	450
	2013	–	–	–	450	–	–	–	–
Regional total	**2011**	**22 298**	**0**	**18 025**	**150 986**	**1 391**	**0**	**23 188**	**32 267**
	2012	**39 151**	**0**	**15 775**	**168 776**	**1 242**	**0**	**21 664**	**32 441**
	2013	**351 956**	**490 302**	**12 813**	**1 628 630**	**1 906**	**2**	**1 297 977**	**221 051**
	2014	**333 253**	**816**	**7 931**	**3 350 198**	**640**	**0**	**7 397 880**	**2 744 624**
	2015	**10 199**	**9 575**	**911**	**566 170**	**727**	**0**	**177 183**	**93 629**

South Asia

Country or territory, by region	Year	Acetone (litres)	Anthranilic acid (kilograms)	Ethyl ether (litres)	Hydrochloric acid (litres)	Methyl ethyl ketone (litres)	Piperidine (litres)	Sulphuric acid (litres)	Toluene (litres)
India	2014	–	–	–	–	110 364	–	–	–
	2015	–	–	–	–	32	–	–	–
Maldives	2011	–	–	–	14	–	–	5	–
Regional total	**2011**	**0**	**0**	**0**	**14**	**0**	**0**	**5**	**0**
	2012	**0**	**0**	**0**	**0**	**0**	**0**	**0**	**0**
	2013	**0**	**0**	**0**	**0**	**0**	**0**	**0**	**0**
	2014	**0**	**0**	**0**	**0**	**110 364**	**0**	**0**	**0**
	2015	**0**	**0**	**0**	**0**	**32**	**0**	**0**	**0**

ANNEXES

Country or territory, by region	Year	Acetone (litres)	Anthranilic acid (kilograms)	Ethyl ether (litres)	Hydrochloric acid (litres)	Methyl ethyl ketone (litres)	Piperidine (litres)	Sulphuric acid (litres)	Toluene (litres)
West Asia									
Afghanistan	2011	–	–	–	120	–	–	–	–
	2012	–	–	–	–	–	–	3 764	–
	2013	174	–	–	4 705	–	–	–	–
	2014	–	–	–	5 317	–	–	19 075	25
	2015	–	–	–	–	–	–	15 900	363
Armenia	2011	○	–	–	○	–	–	○	–
	2012	–	–	–	○	–	–	–	–
	2013	–	–	○	○	–	–	–	–
	2014	–	–	○	–	–	–	–	–
Kazakhstan	2011	78	–	–	10 707	–	–	698	–
	2012	1	–	–	1 600	–	–	913	–
Kyrgyzstan	2012	–	–	–	98	–	–	3 703	–
	2013	–	–	–	–	–	–	4 386	–
	2014	–	–	–	535	–	–	12 756	–
	2015	–	–	–	404	–	–	8 144	–
Lebanon	2011	–	–	○	–	–	–	–	–
	2012	13	–	2 358	–	–	–	–	–
	2014	32	–	43	10	–	–	–	–
Pakistan	2012	–	–	–	–	–	–	326	–
	2013	–	–	–	925	–	–	326	–

PRECURSORS

Country or territory, by region	Year	Acetone (litres)	Anthranilic acid (kilograms)	Ethyl ether (litres)	Hydrochloric acid (litres)	Methyl ethyl ketone (litres)	Piperidine (litres)	Sulphuric acid (litres)	Toluene (litres)
Qatar	2014	–	–	–	9 996	–	–	27 367	–
	2015	–	–	–	30	–	–	–	–
	2013	565	–	–	407 363	–	°	443 814	597
Tajikistan	2011	–	–	–	–	–	–	6 803	–
	2012	–	–	–	–	14	–	1	–
Turkey	2011	3	–	–	–	–	–	–	–
Uzbekistan	2011	274	–	–	40	–	–	2 540	–
	2014	–	–	–	–	–	–	1 610	–
	2015	10 500	–	–	–	–	–	7 800	–
Regional total	**2011**	**354**	**0**	**0**	**10 867**	**0**	**0**	**10 040**	**0**
	2012	**14**	**0**	**2 358**	**1 698**	**14**	**0**	**8 707**	**0**
	2013	**739**	**0**	**0**	**412 993**	**0**	**0**	**448 526**	**597**
	2014	**32**	**0**	**43**	**15 859**	**0**	**0**	**60 809**	**25**
	2015	**10 500**	**0**	**0**	**434**	**0**	**0**	**31 844**	**363**
Europe									
States not members of the European Union									
Belarus	2013	–	–	–	–	–	–	10 751	–
	2014	94	–	–	–	–	–	–	–
	2015	2 931	–	–	16 329	–	–	–	1 104

ANNEXES

Country or territory, by region	Year	Acetone (litres)	Anthranilic acid (kilograms)	Ethyl ether (litres)	Hydrochloric acid (litres)	Methyl ethyl ketone (litres)	Piperidine (litres)	Sulphuric acid (litres)	Toluene (litres)
Norway									
	2013	1	–	–	○	–	–	–	–
	2015	–	–	–	–	–	–	–	○
Russian Federation									
	2011	–	–	–	48	–	–	66	–
	2012	–	–	–	26	–	–	91 433	–
	2013	–	–	–	5	–	–	15	–
	2014	–	–	–	1	–	–	7	–
	2015	–	–	–	1	–	–	14	–
Republic of Moldova									
	2015	–	–	–	2	–	–	○	–
Serbia									
	2012	–	–	–	–	–	–	–	20
Ukraine									
	2011	1 821	–	555	24 608	1 706	–	281 755	4 245
	2012	10 324	–	9 216	2 211	720	–	3 302	20 089
	2013	1 163	–	–	3 053	–	–	631	602
	2015	4 275	–	–	182	–	–	35	24 180
States members of the European Union									
Austria									
	2011	○	–	1	○	–	–	2	–
	2012	–	–	–	–	18	–	–	1
	2013	3	–	○	9	–	–	–	6
	2014	1	–	–	18	–	–	121	73
	2015	7	–	–	9	–	–	5	4

PRECURSORS

Country or territory, by region	Year	Acetone (litres)	Anthranilic acid (kilograms)	Ethyl ether (litres)	Hydrochloric acid (litres)	Methyl ethyl ketone (litres)	Piperidine (litres)	Sulphuric acid (litres)	Toluene (litres)
Belgium	2011	602	–	–	839	–	–	3 733	–
	2012	52	–	–	735	–	–	30	–
Bulgaria	2011	–	–	3	34	–	–	20	–
	2012	5	–	2	2	–	–	10	–
	2013	–	–	–	9	–	–	2	12
Cyprus	2014	–	–	–	∘	–	–	–	–
Czechia[c]	2014	1 380	–	–	822	–	–	–	1 571
Estonia	2011	–	–	–	–	–	–	3	10
	2012	–	–	5	–	–	–	27	–
	2013	–	–	–	1	–	–	1	–
	2015	–	–	–	∘	–	–	∘	–
Finland	2011	6	–	–	23	–	–	1	1
	2012	–	–	–	–	–	–	3	–
France	2012	–	–	1	–	3 019	–	1	1
Germany	2011	17	–	5	77	63	–	8	9
	2012	94	–	97	717	–	–	71	1 164
	2013	12	–	∘	15	1	–	48	20

ANNEXES

Country or territory, by region	Year	Acetone (litres)	Anthranilic acid (kilograms)	Ethyl ether (litres)	Hydrochloric acid (litres)	Methyl ethyl ketone (litres)	Piperidine (litres)	Sulphuric acid (litres)	Toluene (litres)
	2014	10	—	—	6	—	—	27	17
	2015	18	—	—	6	—	—	32	2
Hungary	2011	37	—	7	11	—	—	4	6
	2012	35	—	7	11	—	—	—	—
	2013	75	—	2	—	—	—	○	—
	2014	12	—	—	○	—	—	○	—
	2015	26	—	—	—	—	—	—	23
Latvia	2012	81	—	○	24	—	—	12	—
Lithuania	2011	—	—	2	—	—	—	—	—
Netherlands	2011	6 485	—	—	8 429	—	—	12 404	—
	2012	1 245	—	—	4 567	—	—	2 020	—
	2013	—	—	—	19 988	—	—	8 165	1
	2014	8 510	—	—	13 825	—	—	6 555	—
	2015	20 887	—	812	20 266	409	—	28 265	465
Poland	2011	58	—	4	45	—	—	58	103
	2012	285	—	—	3 575	—	—	148	15
	2013	—	—	—	40	—	—	1 436	—
	2014	130	—	—	8	—	—	11	196
	2015	—	—	—	121	—	—	57	.7

PRECURSORS

Country or territory, by region	Year	Acetone (litres)	Anthranilic acid (kilograms)	Ethyl ether (litres)	Hydrochloric acid (litres)	Methyl ethyl ketone (litres)	Piperidine (litres)	Sulphuric acid (litres)	Toluene (litres)
Portugal	2012	0	–	–	–	–	–	–	–
	2013	3	–	–	2	–	–	1	–
	2015	64	–	5	9	–	–	–	–
Romania	2012	3	–	–	–	–	–	–	–
Slovakia	2011	3	–	–	13	–	–	–	28
	2012	1	–	–	2	–	–	–	20
	2013	–	–	–	8	–	–	–	6
	2014	1	–	1	10	–	–	3	18
	2015	–	–	–	1	–	–	–	43
Spain	2011	1	–	0	1	1	–	1	0
	2012	425	–	287	990	123	50	30	33
	2013	1 190	–	297	490	2 197	–	1 086 979	11 511 987
	2014	85	–	20	159	1	–	1	2
	2015	941	–	78	4 412	1 061	–	444	1
Sweden	2011	–	0	–	–	–	–	–	–
United Kingdom	2012	–	–	21	–	385	–	–	–
	2013	–	–	–	–	–	–	20	–
Regional total	**2011**	**9 028**	**0**	**574**	**34 127**	**1 770**	**0**	**298 054**	**4 401**
	2012	**12 549**	**0**	**9 635**	**12 859**	**4 266**	**50**	**97 087**	**21 343**
	2013	**2 447**	**0**	**299**	**23 621**	**2 197**	**0**	**1 108 049**	**11 512 633**

Country or territory, by region	Year	Acetone (litres)	Anthranilic acid (kilograms)	Ethyl ether (litres)	Hydrochloric acid (litres)	Methyl ethyl ketone (litres)	Piperidine (litres)	Sulphuric acid (litres)	Toluene (litres)
	2014	10 221	0	21	14 851	1	0	6 724	1 878
	2015	29 148	0	897	41 338	1 470	0	28 851	25 829
Oceania									
Australia									
	2011	51	–	1	88	–	–	9	14
	2012	130	–	–	112	16	–	62	83
	2015	–	2	–	–	–	–	–	–
New Zealand									
	2011	203	–	–	308	26	–	28	476
	2012	93	–	–	137	–	–	10	682
	2013	108	–	–	263	13	–	74	835
	2015	45	–	–	313	–	–	46	140
Regional total									
	2011	254	0	1	396	26	0	37	490
	2012	223	0	0	249	16	0	72	765
	2013	108	0	0	263	13	0	74	835
	2014	0	0	0	0	0	0	0	0
	2015	45	2	0	313	0	0	46	140
World total									
	2011	696 666	0	20 970	679 785	7 343	12	2 040 787	142 307
	2012	986 216	0	60 854	504 165	11 069	257	512 447	126 932
	2013	1 038 128	490 302	43 708	2 332 546	9 264	59	4 146 274	11 749 436
	2014	937 648	816	11 585	3 572 000	118 776	57	7 888 787	2 946 513
	2015	989 743	9 577	26 368	1 472 951	2 628	0	930 335	285 170

[a] The exact quantity of the seizures was not specified.
[b] For statistical purposes, the data for China do not include those for the Hong Kong Special Administrative Region (SAR) of China and the Macao SAR of China.
[c] Since 17 May 2016, "Czechia" has replaced "Czech Republic" as the short name used in the United Nations.

Annex IX

Submission of information by Governments on licit trade in, uses of and requirements for substances in Tables I and II of the 1988 Convention for the years 2011-2015

Governments of the countries and territories indicated have provided information on licit trade in, uses of and requirements for substances in Tables I and II of the United Nations Convention against Illicit Traffic in Narcotic Drugs and Psychotropic Substances of 1988 on form D for the years 2011-2015. That information was requested in accordance with Economic and Social Council resolution 1995/20. Details may be made available on a case-by-case basis, subject to confidentiality of data.

Notes: The names of non-metropolitan territories and special administrative regions are in italics.
"X" signifies that relevant information was submitted on form D.

Country or territory	2011		2012		2013		2014		2015	
	Trade	Uses and/or requirements	Trade	Uses and/or requirements	Trade	Uses and/or requirements	Trade	Uses and/or requirements	Trade	Uses and/or requirements
Afghanistan			X	X	X	X	X	X	X	X
Albania	X	X	X	X	X	X	X	X	X	X
Algeria	X	X	X	X	X	X	X	X		
Andorra			X	X	X	X				X
Angola										
Anguilla										
Antigua and Barbuda										
Argentina	X	X	X	X	X	X	X	X	X	X
Armenia	X	X	X	X	X	X	X	X	X	
Aruba										
Ascension Island										
Australia	X	X	X	X	X	X	X	X	X	X
Austria[a]	X	X	X	X	X	X	X	X	X	X
Azerbaijan	X	X	X	X	X	X	X	X	X	X
Bahamas										
Bahrain							X	X	X	X
Bangladesh	X	X	X	X	X	X	X	X	X	X
Barbados					X	X				
Belarus	X	X	X	X	X	X	X	X	X	X
Belgium[a]	X	X	X	X	X	X	X	X	X	X
Belize					X	X				
Benin	X	X	X	X	X	X	X	X	X	X
Bermuda										
Bhutan	X	X	X	X			X	X	X	X
Bolivia (Plurinational State of)	X	X	X	X	X	X	X	X	X	X
Bosnia and Herzegovina	X	X	X	X	X	X	X	X	X	X

ANNEXES

Country or territory	2011 Trade	2011 Uses and/or require- ments	2012 Trade	2012 Uses and/or require- ments	2013 Trade	2013 Uses and/or require- ments	2014 Trade	2014 Uses and/or require- ments	2015 Trade	2015 Uses and/or require- ments
Botswana										
Brazil			X	X	X	X	X	X	X	X
British Virgin Islands										
Brunei Darussalam	X	X	X	X	X	X	X	X	X	X
Bulgaria[a]	X		X	X	X	X	X	X	X	X
Burkina Faso	X	X								
Burundi									X	X
Cabo Verde							X	X	X	X
Cambodia			X		X	X		X		
Cameroon	X		X	X			X	X		
Canada	X	X	X	X	X	X	X	X	X	X
Cayman Islands										
Central African Republic										
Chad										
Chile	X	X	X	X	X	X	X	X	X	X
China	X	X	X	X	X	X	X	X	X	
China, Hong Kong SAR			X	X	X	X				
China, Macao SAR			X	X	X	X	X	X		
Christmas Island	X	X			X				X	X
Cocos (Keeling) Islands									X	X
Colombia	X	X	X	X	X	X	X	X	X	X
Comoros										
Congo										
Cook Islands	X	X								
Costa Rica	X	X	X	X	X	X	X	X	X	X
Côte d'Ivoire	X	X	X	X	X	X	X	X		
Croatia[a]	X		X	X	X	X	X	X	X	X
Cuba	X	X								
Curaçao	X	X	X	X	X	X	X	X	X	X
Cyprus[a]	X	X	X	X	X	X	X	X	X	X
Czechia[a,b]	X	X	X	X	X	X	X	X	X	X
Democratic People's Republic of Korea		X		X		X				X
Democratic Republic of the Congo	X	X	X	X	X		X		X	
Denmark[a]	X		X	X	X		X	X	X	X
Djibouti										
Dominica										
Dominican Republic					X	X	X	X		
Ecuador	X	X	X	X	X	X	X	X	X	X

PRECURSORS

Country or territory	2011		2012		2013		2014		2015	
	Trade	Uses and/or requirements	Trade	Uses and/or requirements	Trade	Uses and/or requirements	Trade	Uses and/or requirements	Trade	Uses and/or requirements
Egypt	X	X	X	X	X	X	X	X	X	X
El Salvador	X	X	X	X	X	X	X	X	X	X
Equatorial Guinea										
Eritrea	X	X	X	X						
Estonia[a]	X	X	X	X		X	X	X	X	X
Ethiopia	X	X	X	X	X	X			X	X
Falkland Islands (Malvinas)	X	X	X	X	X	X	X	X	X	X
Fiji	X	X								
Finland[a]	X	X	X	X	X	X	X	X	X	X
France[a]	X	X	X	X	X	X	X	X	X	X
French Polynesia									X	X
Gabon										
Gambia					X	X				
Georgia	X	X	X	X	X	X	X	X	X	X
Germany[a]	X	X	X	X	X	X	X	X	X	X
Ghana	X	X	X	X	X	X	X	X	X	X
Gibraltar										
Greece[a]	X	X	X	X	X	X	X	X	X	X
Grenada										
Guatemala			X	X	X	X	X	X	X	X
Guinea										
Guinea-Bissau										
Guyana							X	X		X
Haiti	X	X			X	X	X	X	X	X
Holy See[c]										
Honduras	X	X	X	X	X	X			X	X
Hungary[a]	X	X	X	X	X	X	X	X	X	X
Iceland	X	X	X	X	X	X	X	X	X	X
India	X	X	X	X	X	X	X	X	X	X
Indonesia	X	X	X	X	X	X	X	X	X	X
Iran (Islamic Republic of)					X	X	X	X	X	X
Iraq	X	X								
Ireland[a]	X	X	X	X	X	X	X	X	X	X
Israel	X	X	X	X	X	X	X	X	X	X
Italy[a]	X	X	X	X	X	X	X	X	X	X
Jamaica					X	X	X	X	X	X
Japan	X	X	X	X	X	X	X	X	X	X
Jordan	X	X	X	X	X	X	X	X	X	X
Kazakhstan	X	X			X	X			X	X

Country or territory	2011 Trade	2011 Uses and/or requirements	2012 Trade	2012 Uses and/or requirements	2013 Trade	2013 Uses and/or requirements	2014 Trade	2014 Uses and/or requirements	2015 Trade	2015 Uses and/or requirements
Kenya									X	X
Kiribati										
Kuwait			X	X	X	X				
Kyrgyzstan	X	X	X	X	X	X	X	X	X	X
Lao People's Democratic Republic	X	X	X	X	X	X	X		X	
Latvia[a]	X	X	X	X	X	X	X	X	X	X
Lebanon	X	X	X	X	X	X	X	X	X	X
Lesotho								X		
Liberia	X									
Libya										
Liechtenstein[d]										
Lithuania[a]	X	X		X	X	X	X	X	X	X
Luxembourg[a]										
Madagascar					X	X	X	X	X	X
Malawi										
Malaysia	X	X	X	X	X	X	X	X	X	X
Maldives	X	X	X	X	X	X				
Mali					X	X				
Malta[a]	X	X		X	X	X	X	X	X	X
Marshall Islands										
Mauritania										
Mauritius	X	X	X	X						
Mexico	X	X	X	X	X	X	X	X	X	X
Micronesia (Federated States of)					X	X				
Monaco[e]										
Mongolia	X		X	X	X				X	X
Montenegro	X	X	X	X	X	X	X	X	X	X
Montserrat			X	X	X	X	X	X	X	X
Morocco	X	X	X	X	X	X	X	X	X	X
Mozambique							X			
Myanmar	X	X	X	X	X	X	X	X	X	X
Namibia										
Nauru										
Nepal					X	X	X	X		
Netherlands[a]	X	X	X	X	X	X	X	X	X	X
New Caledonia										
New Zealand	X	X	X	X	X	X			X	X
Nicaragua	X	X	X	X	X	X	X	X	X	X

PRECURSORS

Country or territory	2011 Trade	2011 Uses and/or requirements	2012 Trade	2012 Uses and/or requirements	2013 Trade	2013 Uses and/or requirements	2014 Trade	2014 Uses and/or requirements	2015 Trade	2015 Uses and/or requirements
Niger										
Nigeria	X	X	X	X	X	X				
Niue										
Norfolk Island									X	X
Norway			X	X	X	X	X	X	X	X
Oman							X	X	X	X
Pakistan	X	X	X	X	X	X	X	X	X	X
Palau										
Panama	X	X	X	X	X	X	X	X	X	X
Papua New Guinea										
Paraguay	X	X								
Peru	X	X	X	X	X	X	X	X	X	X
Philippines	X	X	X	X	X	X	X	X	X	X
Poland[a]	X	X	X	X	X	X	X	X	X	X
Portugal[a]	X		X		X	X	X	X	X	X
Qatar	X	X			X	X				
Republic of Korea	X	X	X	X	X	X	X	X	X	X
Republic of Moldova	X	X	X	X	X	X	X	X	X	X
Romania[a]	X	X	X	X	X	X	X	X	X	X
Russian Federation	X	X	X	X	X	X	X	X	X	X
Rwanda									X	X
Saint Helena	X	X								
Saint Kitts and Nevis										
Saint Lucia			X	X	X	X	X	X	X	X
Saint Vincent and the Grenadines			X	X	X	X	X	X	X	X
Samoa			X	X						
San Marino[c]										
Sao Tome and Principe										
Saudi Arabia	X		X		X	X	X	X	X	X
Senegal					X	X	X	X	X	X
Serbia	X	X	X	X	X	X				
Seychelles	X	X	X	X						
Sierra Leone										
Singapore	X	X	X	X	X	X	X	X	X	X
Sint Maarten										
Slovakia[a]	X	X	X	X	X	X	X	X	X	X
Slovenia[a]	X	X	X	X	X	X	X	X	X	X
Solomon Islands										

ANNEXES

Country or territory	2011 Trade	2011 Uses and/or requirements	2012 Trade	2012 Uses and/or requirements	2013 Trade	2013 Uses and/or requirements	2014 Trade	2014 Uses and/or requirements	2015 Trade	2015 Uses and/or requirements
Somalia										
South Africa					X	X			X	X
South Sudan[f]										
Spain[a]	X	X	X	X	X	X	X	X	X	X
Sri Lanka	X	X	X	X	X	X	X		X	
Sudan							X	X	X	
Suriname										
Swaziland										
Sweden[a]	X	X	X	X	X	X	X	X	X	X
Switzerland	X	X	X	X	X	X	X	X	X	X
Syrian Arab Republic			X	X	X	X	X		X	
Tajikistan	X	X	X	X	X	X			X	X
Thailand	X	X	X	X	X	X	X	X	X	X
The former Yugoslav Republic of Macedonia										
Timor-Leste										
Togo			X	X						
Tonga										
Trinidad and Tobago	X	X	X	X	X	X	X	X	X	X
Tristan da Cunha										
Tunisia	X	X	X	X	X	X	X	X	X	X
Turkey	X	X	X	X	X	X	X	X	X	X
Turkmenistan			X	X	X	X	X	X	X	X
Turks and Caicos Islands										
Tuvalu	X	X								
Uganda	X	X	X	X	X	X	X	X	X	
Ukraine	X	X	X	X	X	X			X	X
United Arab Emirates	X	X	X	X	X	X	X	X		
United Kingdom[a]	X	X	X	X		X	X	X	X	X
United Republic of Tanzania	X	X	X	X	X	X	X	X	X	X
United States of America	X	X	X	X	X	X	X	X	X	X
Uruguay	X	X	X	X	X	X	X	X	X	X
Uzbekistan	X	X	X	X	X	X	X	X	X	X
Vanuatu	X	X								
Venezuela (Bolivarian Republic of)	X	X	X	X	X	X	X	X	X	X
Viet Nam	X	X	X	X	X	X	X	X	X	X
Wallis and Futuna Islands										
Yemen	X	X	X	X						
Zambia							X	X		

PRECURSORS

Country or territory	2011 Trade	2011 Uses and/or require- ments	2012 Trade	2012 Uses and/or require- ments	2013 Trade	2013 Uses and/or require- ments	2014 Trade	2014 Uses and/or require- ments	2015 Trade	2015 Uses and/or require- ments
Zimbabwe		X			X	X	X	X	X	X
Total number of governments that submitted form D	120	114	120	120	129	128	118	115	123	118
Total number of governments requested to provide information	213	213	213	213	213	213	213	213	213	213

[a] State member of the European Union.
[b] Since 17 May 2016, "Czechia" has replaced "Czech Republic" as the short name used in the United Nations.
[c] The Government of Italy includes on form D licit trade data for the Holy See and San Marino.
[d] The Government of Switzerland includes on form D licit trade data for Liechtenstein.
[e] The Government of France includes on form D licit trade data for Monaco.
[f] By its resolution 65/308 of 14 July 2011, the General Assembly decided to admit South Sudan to membership in the United Nations.

Annex X

Governments that have requested pre-export notifications pursuant to article 12, paragraph 10 (a), of the 1988 Convention

1. Governments of all exporting countries and territories are reminded that it is an obligation to provide pre-export notifications to Governments that have requested them pursuant to article 12, paragraph 10 (a), of the United Nations Convention against Illicit Traffic in Narcotic Drugs and Psychotropic Substances of 1988, which provides that:

> "upon request to the Secretary-General by the interested Party, each Party from whose territory a substance in Table I is to be exported shall ensure that, prior to such export, the following information is supplied by its competent authorities to the competent authorities of the importing country:
>
> "(i) Name and address of the exporter and importer and, when available, the consignee;
>
> "(ii) Name of the substance in Table I;
>
> "(iii) Quantity of the substance to be exported;
>
> "(iv) Expected point of entry and expected date of dispatch;
>
> "(v) Any other information which is mutually agreed upon by the Parties."

2. Governments that have requested pre-export notifications are listed in the table below in alphabetical order, followed by the substance (or substances) for which pre-export notifications were requested, and the date of notification of the request transmitted by the Secretary-General to Governments.

3. The information is current as at 4 November 2016.

Notifying Government	Substances for which pre-export notifications have been requested	Date of communication to Governments by the Secretary-General
Afghanistan[a]	All substances included in Tables I and II	13 July 2010
Algeria[a]	All substances included in Tables I and II	10 October 2013
Antigua and Barbuda[a]	All substances included in Tables I and II	5 May 2000
Argentina	All substances included in Table I	19 November 1999
Armenia[a]	All substances included in Tables I and II[b,c]	4 July 2013
Australia[a]	All substances included in Tables I and II	12 February 2010
Austria	All substances included in Table I	19 May 2000[d]
Azerbaijan[a]	All substances included in Tables I and II	21 January 2011
Bangladesh[a]	All substances included in Tables I and II	12 May 2015
Barbados[a]	All substances included in Tables I and II[b,c]	24 October 2013
Belarus[e]	Acetic anhydride, ephedrine, potassium permanganate and pseudoephedrine	12 October 2000
Belgium	All substances included in Table I	19 May 2000

Notifying Government	Substances for which pre-export notifications have been requested	Date of communication to Governments by the Secretary-General
Benin[a]	All substances included in Tables I and II	4 February 2000
Bolivia (Plurinational State of)[a]	Acetic anhydride, acetone, ethyl ether, hydrochloric acid, potassium permanganate and sulphuric acid	12 November 2001
Brazil[a]	All substances included in Tables I and II	15 October and 15 December 1999
Bulgaria	All substances included in Table I	19 May 2000[d]
Canada[a]	All substances included in Tables I and II	31 October 2005
Cayman Islands[a]	All substances included in Tables I and II	7 September 1998
Chile[a]	All substances included in Tables I and II	19 October 2012
China	Acetic anhydride	20 October 2000
China, Hong Kong SAR[a]	All substances included in Tables I and II	28 December 2012
China, Macao SAR[a]	All substances included in Tables I and II	28 December 2012
Colombia[a]	All substances included in Tables I and II	14 October 1998
Costa Rica[a]	All substances included in Tables I and II	27 September 1999
Côte d'Ivoire[a]	All substances included in Tables I and II	26 June 2013
Croatia	All substances included in Table I	19 May 2000[d]
Cyprus	All substances included in Table I	19 May 2000[d]
Czechia[g]	All substances included in Table I	19 May 2000[d]
Denmark	All substances included in Table I	19 May 2000[d]
Dominican Republic[a]	All substances included in Tables I and II	11 September 2002
Ecuador[a]	All substances included in Tables I and II	1 August 1996
Egypt[a]	All substances included in Table I and acetone	3 December 2004
El Salvador[a]	All substances included in Tables I and II	29 July 2010
Estonia	All substances included in Table I	19 May 2000
Ethiopia[a]	All substances included in Tables I and II	17 December 1999
Finland	All substances included in Table I	19 May 2000[d]
France	All substances included in Table I	19 May 2000[d]
Georgia[a]	All substances included in Tables I and II	7 September 2016
Germany	All substances included in Table I	19 May 2000[d]
Ghana[a]	All substances included in Tables I and II	26 February 2010
Greece	All substances included in Table I	19 May 2000[d]
Haiti[a]	All substances included in Tables I and II	20 June 2002
Hungary	All substances included in Table I	19 May 2000[d]
India[a]	All substances included in Tables I and II	23 March 2000
Indonesia[a]	Acetic anhydride, N-acetylanthranilic acid, anthranilic acid, ephedrine, ergometrine, ergotamine, isosafrole, 3,4-methylenedioxyphenyl-2-propanone, phenylacetic acid, 1-phenyl-2-propanone, piperonal, pseudoephedrine and safrole	18 February 2000

Notifying Government	Substances for which pre-export notifications have been requested	Date of communication to Governments by the Secretary-General
Iraq[a]	All substances included in Tables I and II[b,c]	31 July 2013
Ireland	All substances included in Table I	19 May 2000[d]
Italy	All substances included in Table I	19 May 2000[d]
Jamaica	All substances included in Table I[b,c]	4 July 2013
Japan	All substances included in Table I	17 December 1999
Jordan[a]	All substances included in Tables I and II	15 December 1999
Kazakhstan[a]	All substances included in Tables I and II	15 August 2003
Kenya[a]	All substances included in Tables I and II[b,c]	10 October 2013
Kyrgyzstan[a]	All substances included in Tables I and II[b,c]	21 October 2013
Latvia	All substances included in Table I	19 May 2000[d]
Lebanon[a]	All substances included in Tables I and II	14 June 2002
Libya[a]	All substances included in Tables I and II[b,c]	21 August 2013
Lithuania	All substances included in Table I	19 May 2000[d]
Luxembourg	All substances included in Table I	19 May 2000[d]
Madagascar[a]	All substances included in Tables I and II	31 March 2003
Malaysia[a]	All substances included in Table I,[b] anthranilic acid, ethyl ether and piperidine	21 August 1998
Maldives[a]	All substances included in Tables I and II	6 April 2005
Malta	All substances included in Table I	19 May 2000[d]
Mexico[a]	All substances included in Tables I and II	6 April 2005
Micronesia (Federal States of)[a]	All substances included in Tables I and II[b,c]	11 February 2014
Myanmar[a]	All substances included in Tables I and II[c]	4 November 2016
Netherlands	All substances included in Table I	19 May 2000[d]
New Zealand[a]	All substances included in Tables I and II[b,c]	3 April 2014
Nicaragua[a]	All substances included in Tables I and II	8 January 2014
Nigeria[a]	All substances included in Tables I and II	28 February 2000
Norway[a]	All substances included in Table I,[c] anthranilic acid, ethyl ether and piperidine	17 December 2013
Oman[a]	All substances included in Tables I and II	16 April 2007
Pakistan[a]	All substances included in Tables I and II	12 November 2001 and 6 March 2013
Panama	Ephedrine, ergometrine, ergotamine, norephedrine and pseudoephedrine	14 August 2013
Paraguay[a]	All substances included in Tables I and II	3 February 2000
Peru[a]	Acetic anhydride, acetone, ephedrine, ergometrine, ergotamine, ethyl ether, hydrochloric acid, lysergic acid, methyl ethyl ketone, norephedrine, potassium permanganate, pseudoephedrine, sulphuric acid and toluene	27 September 1999
Philippines[a]	All substances included in Tables I and II	16 April 1999
Poland	All substances included in Table I	19 May 2000[d]

Notifying Government	Substances for which pre-export notifications have been requested	Date of communication to Governments by the Secretary-General
Portugal	All substances included in Table I	19 May 2000[d]
Qatar[a]	All substances included in Tables I and II[b,c]	16 July 2013
Republic of Korea[a]	All substances included in Table I and acetone	3 June 2008
Republic of Moldova[a]	All substances included in Tables I and II[b,c]	29 December 1998 and 8 November 2013
Romania	All substances included in Table I	19 May 2000[d]
Russian Federation[a]	Acetic anhydride, ephedrine, ergometrine, ergotamine, 3,4-methylenedioxyphenyl-2-propanone, norephedrine, phenylacetic acid, 1-phenyl-2-propanone, potassium permanganate, pseudoephedrine and all substances included in Table II	21 February 2000
Saint Vincent and the Grenadines[a]	All substances included in Tables I and II[b,c]	16 July 2013
Saudi Arabia[a]	All substances included in Tables I and II	18 October 1998
Sierra Leone[a]	All substances included in Tables I and II[b,c]	5 July 2013
Singapore	All substances included in Table I	5 May 2000
Slovakia	All substances included in Table I	19 May 2000[d]
Slovenia	All substances included in Table I	19 May 2000[d]
South Africa[a]	All substances included in Table I and anthranilic acid	11 August 1999
Spain	All substances included in Table I	19 May 2000[d]
Sri Lanka	All substances included in Table I	19 November 1999
Sudan[a]	All substances included in Tables I and II	6 May 2015
Sweden	All substances included in Table I	19 May 2000[d]
Switzerland	All substances included in Table I	25 March 2013
Syrian Arab Republic[a]	All substances included in Tables I and II	24 October 2013
Tajikistan[a]	All substances included in Tables I and II	7 February 2000
Thailand[a]	All substances included in Table I (except potassium permanganate) and anthranilic acid[b]	18 October 2010
Togo[a]	All substances included in Tables I and II	6 August 2013
Tonga[a]	All substances included in Tables I and II[b,c]	4 July 2013
Trinidad and Tobago[a]	All substances included in Tables I and II[b,c]	15 August 2013
Turkey[a]	All substances included in Tables I and II	2 November 1995
Uganda[a]	All substances included in Tables I and II	6 May 2014
United Arab Emirates[a]	All substances included in Tables I[b] and II	26 September 1995
United Kingdom	All substances included in Table I	19 May 2000[d]
United Republic of Tanzania[a]	All substances included in Tables I and II	10 December 2002
United States of America	Acetic anhydride, ephedrine and pseudoephedrine	2 June 1995 and 19 January 2001
Uruguay[a]	All substances included in Tables I and II	30 December 2015
Venezuela (Bolivarian Republic of)[a]	All substances included in Tables I and II	27 March 2000

Notifying Government	Substances for which pre-export notifications have been requested	Date of communication to Governments by the Secretary-General
Yemen[a]	All substances included in Tables I and II	6 May 2014
Zimbabwe[a]	All substances included in Tables I and II[b,c]	4 July 2013
European Union (on behalf of all its States members)[f]	All substances included in Table I	19 May 2000[d]

Note: The names of territories are in italics.

[a] The Secretary-General has informed all Governments of the request of the notifying Government to receive a pre-export notification for some or all substances listed in Table II of the 1988 Convention as well.

[b] Government requested to receive pre-export notifications for pharmaceutical preparations containing ephedrine and pseudoephedrine as well.

[c] Governments requested to receive pre-export notifications for safrole-rich oils as well.

[d] On 19 May 2000, the Secretary-General communicated to Governments the request by the European Commission, on behalf of the State members of the European Union, to receive pre-export notifications for the indicated substances.

[e] Not yet notified by the Secretary-General as, in a subsequent communication, the Government of Belarus requested the Secretary-General to suspend such notification until a national mechanism to receive and process pre-export notifications is established.

[f] Austria, Belgium, Bulgaria, Croatia, Cyprus, Czechia, Denmark, Estonia, Finland, France, Germany, Greece, Hungary, Ireland, Italy, Latvia, Lithuania, Luxembourg, Malta, Netherlands, Poland, Portugal, Romania, Slovakia, Slovenia, Spain, Sweden and the United Kingdom of Great Britain and Northern Ireland.

[g] Since 17 May 2016, "Czechia" has replaced "Czech Republic" as the short name used in the United Nations.

Annex XI

Licit uses of the substances in Tables I and II of the 1988 Convention

Knowledge of the most common licit uses of substances in Tables I and II of the United Nations Convention against Illicit Traffic in Narcotic Drugs and Psychotropic Substances of 1988, including the processes and end products in which the substances may be used, is essential to the verification of the legitimacy of orders or shipments. The most common licit uses of those substances reported to the International Narcotics Control Board are as follows:

Substance	Licit uses
Acetic anhydride	Acetylating and dehydrating agent used in the chemical and pharmaceutical industries for the manufacture of cellulose acetate, for textile sizing agents and cold bleaching activators, for polishing metals and for the production of brake fluids, dyes and explosives
Acetone	Common solvent in the chemical and pharmaceutical industries; used in the production of lubricating oils and as an intermediate in the manufacture of chloroform and in the manufacture of plastics, paints, varnishes and cosmetics
N-Acetylanthranilic acid	Used in the manufacture of pharmaceuticals, plastics and fine chemicals
Anthranilic acid	Chemical intermediate used in the manufacture of dyes, pharmaceuticals and perfumes; also used in the preparation of bird and insect repellents
Ephedrine	Used in the manufacture of bronchodilators (cough medicines)
Ergometrine	Used in the treatment of migraine and as an oxytocic in obstetrics
Ergotamine	Used in the treatment of migraine and as an oxytocic in obstetrics
Ethyl ether	Commonly used solvent in chemical laboratories and in the chemical and pharmaceutical industries; mainly used as an extractant for fats, oils, waxes and resins; also used for the manufacture of munitions, plastics and perfumes and, in medicine, as a general anaesthetic
Hydrochloric acid	Used in the production of chlorides and hydrochlorides, for the neutralization of basic systems and as a catalyst and solvent in organic synthesis
Isosafrole	Used in the manufacture of piperonal; to modify "oriental perfumes"; to strengthen soap perfumes; in small quantities, together with methyl salicylate, in root beer and sarsaparilla flavours; and as a pesticide
Lysergic acid	Used in organic synthesis
3,4-Methylenedioxyphenyl-2-propanone	Used in the manufacture of piperonal and other perfume components
Methyl ethyl ketone	Common solvent; used in the manufacture of coatings, solvents, degreasing agents, lacquers, resins and smokeless powders
Norephedrine	Used in the manufacture of nasal decongestants and appetite suppressants

Substance	Licit uses
Phenylacetic acid	Used in the chemical and pharmaceutical industries for the manufacture of phenylacetate esters, amphetamine and some derivatives; also used for the synthesis of penicillins and in fragrance applications and cleaning solutions
alpha-Phenylacetoacetonitrile	None, except — in small amounts — for research, development and laboratory analytical purposes
1-Phenyl-2-propanone	Used in the chemical and pharmaceutical industries for the manufacture of amphetamine, methamphetamine and some derivatives; also used for the synthesis of propylhexedrine
Piperidine	Commonly used solvent and reagent in chemical laboratories and in the chemical and pharmaceutical industries; also used in the manufacture of rubber products and plastics
Piperonal	Used in perfumery, in cherry and vanilla flavours, in organic synthesis and as a component for mosquito repellent
Potassium permanganate	Important reagent in analytical and synthetic organic chemistry; used in bleaching applications, disinfectants, antibacterials and antifungal agents and in water purification
Pseudoephedrine	Used in the manufacture of bronchodilators and nasal decongestants
Safrole	Used in perfumery, for example in the manufacture of piperonal, and for denaturing fats in soap manufacture
Sulphuric acid	Used in the production of sulphates; as an acidic oxidizer; as a dehydrating and purifying agent; for the neutralization of alkaline solutions; as a catalyst in organic synthesis; in the manufacture of fertilizers, explosives, dyestuffs and paper; and as a component of drain and metal cleaners, anti-rust compounds and automobile battery fluids
Toluene	Industrial solvent; used in the manufacture of explosives, dyes, coatings and other organic substances and as a gasoline additive

About the International Narcotics Control Board

The International Narcotics Control Board (INCB) is an independent and quasi-judicial control organ, established by treaty, for monitoring the implementation of the international drug control treaties. It had predecessors under the former drug control treaties as far back as the time of the League of Nations.

Composition

INCB consists of 13 members who are elected by the Economic and Social Council and who serve in their personal capacity, not as government representatives. Three members with medical, pharmacological or pharmaceutical experience are elected from a list of persons nominated by the World Health Organization (WHO) and 10 members are elected from a list of persons nominated by Governments. Members of the Board are persons who, by their competence, impartiality and disinterestedness, command general confidence. The Council, in consultation with INCB, makes all arrangements necessary to ensure the full technical independence of the Board in carrying out its functions. INCB has a secretariat that assists it in the exercise of its treaty-related functions. The INCB secretariat is an administrative entity of the United Nations Office on Drugs and Crime, but it reports solely to the Board on matters of substance. INCB closely collaborates with the Office in the framework of arrangements approved by the Council in its resolution 1991/48. INCB also cooperates with other international bodies concerned with drug control, including not only the Council and its Commission on Narcotic Drugs, but also the relevant specialized agencies of the United Nations, particularly WHO. It also cooperates with bodies outside the United Nations system, especially the International Criminal Police Organization (INTERPOL) and the World Customs Organization.

Functions

The functions of INCB are laid down in the following treaties: Single Convention on Narcotic Drugs of 1961 as amended by the 1972 Protocol; Convention on Psychotropic Substances of 1971; and United Nations Convention against Illicit Traffic in Narcotic Drugs and Psychotropic Substances of 1988. Broadly speaking, INCB deals with the following:

(a) As regards the licit manufacture of, trade in and use of drugs, INCB endeavours, in cooperation with Governments, to ensure that adequate supplies of drugs are available for medical and scientific uses and that the diversion of drugs from licit sources to illicit channels does not occur. INCB also monitors Governments' control over chemicals used in the illicit manufacture of drugs and assists them in preventing the diversion of those chemicals into the illicit traffic;

(b) As regards the illicit manufacture of, trafficking in and use of drugs, INCB identifies weaknesses in national and international control systems and contributes to correcting such situations. INCB is also responsible for assessing chemicals used in the illicit manufacture of drugs, in order to determine whether they should be placed under international control.

In the discharge of its responsibilities, INCB:

(a) Administers a system of estimates for narcotic drugs and a voluntary assessment system for psychotropic substances and monitors licit activities involving drugs through a statistical returns system, with a view to assisting Governments in achieving, inter alia, a balance between supply and demand;

(b) Monitors and promotes measures taken by Governments to prevent the diversion of substances frequently used in the illicit manufacture of narcotic drugs and psychotropic substances and assesses such substances to determine whether there is a need for changes in the scope of control of Tables I and II of the 1988 Convention;

(c) Analyses information provided by Governments, United Nations bodies, specialized agencies or other competent international organizations, with a view to ensuring that the provisions of the international drug control treaties are adequately carried out by Governments, and recommends remedial measures;

(d) Maintains a permanent dialogue with Governments to assist them in complying with their obligations under the international drug control treaties and, to that end, recommends, where appropriate, technical or financial assistance to be provided.

INCB is called upon to ask for explanations in the event of apparent violations of the treaties, to propose appropriate remedial measures to Governments that are not fully applying the provisions of the treaties or are encountering difficulties in applying them and, where necessary, to assist Governments in overcoming such difficulties. If, however, INCB notes that the measures necessary to remedy a serious situation have not been taken, it may call the matter to the attention of the parties concerned, the Commission on Narcotic Drugs and the Economic and Social Council. As a last resort, the treaties empower INCB to recommend to parties that they stop importing drugs from a defaulting country, exporting drugs to it or both. In all cases, INCB acts in close cooperation with Governments.

INCB assists national administrations in meeting their obligations under the conventions. To that end, it proposes and participates in regional training seminars and programmes for drug control administrators.

Reports

The international drug control treaties require INCB to prepare an annual report on its work. The annual report contains an analysis of the drug control situation worldwide so that Governments are kept aware of existing and potential situations that may endanger the objectives of the international drug control treaties. INCB draws the attention of Governments to gaps and weaknesses in national control and in treaty compliance; it also makes suggestions and recommendations for improvements at both the national and international levels. The annual report is based on information provided by Governments to INCB, United Nations entities and other organizations. It also uses information provided through other international organizations, such as INTERPOL and the World Customs Organization, as well as regional organizations.

The annual report of INCB is supplemented by detailed technical reports. They contain data on the licit movement of narcotic drugs and psychotropic substances required for medical and scientific purposes, together with an analysis of those data by INCB. Those data are required for the proper functioning of the system of control over the licit movement of narcotic drugs and psychotropic substances, including preventing their diversion to illicit channels. Moreover, under the provisions of article 12 of the 1988 Convention, INCB reports annually to the Commission on Narcotic Drugs on the implementation of that article. That report, which gives an account of the results of the monitoring of precursors and of the chemicals frequently used in the illicit manufacture of narcotic drugs and psychotropic substances, is also published as a supplement to the annual report.